100 Biohacks for Optimal Health and Wellness

Contents

Introduction: Unleashing Human Potential

In an era defined by scientific innovation, the quest for human optimization has taken on an entirely new dimension. We live in a time when individuals are not merely content with the status quo of their health and performance; they aspire to push beyond perceived limits and unlock the full potential of their bodies and minds. This unrelenting pursuit of self-improvement has given birth to a movement known as biohacking.

Welcome to a journey that will take you deep into the heart of biohacking, a field that encapsulates the art and science of enhancing our physical, mental, and emotional well-being through a blend of self-experimentation, data-driven insights, and cutting-edge technologies. In the pages that follow, we will embark on a profound exploration of biohacking's principles, practices, pioneers, and potential.

Biohacking, in its essence, is a testament to the indomitable human spirit—the innate drive to evolve, adapt, and transcend limitations. It's a movement that champions the idea that we can take charge of our own biology, not as passive observers but as active architects of our health and destiny.

This book is not a mere observer's account of the biohacking phenomenon; it is your comprehensive guide, your passport to understanding the intricacies of this dynamic field. Whether you are entirely new to the world of biohacking or a seasoned enthusiast, these pages will offer something for every curious mind.

We will start by defining biohacking and establishing its core principles, highlighting how it has evolved into a formidable movement. We will explore the notion that the human body is a complex, interconnected system, setting the stage for our journey into the various facets of self-improvement.

Throughout these chapters, we will dissect the importance of systems thinking, the delicate balance of homeostasis, and the art of self-experimentation. We will delve into the role of data in biohacking, the ways technology aids us in our quest for self-optimization, and the profound impact of nutrition, sleep, and exercise on our well-being.

But biohacking is not merely a collection of practices; it is a cultural movement driven by pioneers who have boldly ventured into uncharted territories, challenging conventions and pushing the boundaries of human potential. In these pages, we will introduce you to these remarkable individuals, share their journeys, and explore their achievements.

You will encounter a treasure trove of over 100 biohacks curated to empower you on your journey of self-improvement. These biohacks encompass a diverse array of practices, techniques, and strategies designed to optimize every facet of your life, from enhancing cognitive function and achieving peak physical performance to extending your healthspan and fostering holistic well-being. With each biohack, you will uncover a wealth of knowledge, data-driven insights, and practical tips that you can integrate into your daily routine, allowing you to unlock the untapped potential of your body and mind.

Whether you seek to improve your sleep quality, refine your nutrition, harness the power of technology, or explore the frontiers of cognitive enhancement, these biohacks are your keys to transformation, offering a roadmap to a healthier, more vibrant, and fully optimized you.

This is not just a book; it is an invitation to embark on a transformative journey—a journey that empowers you to be the author of your own health and well-being. As we journey through the uncharted terrain of biohacking, we invite you to explore, to question, and to embrace the potential that lies within you.

It's time to unlock your full potential—to unleash the biohacker within. Welcome to the world of biohacking.

Definition of Biohacking

Biohacking is the art and science of pushing the boundaries of human potential. It's about seizing control of your own biology and forging a path to optimized health and peak performance. This chapter introduces the fundamental concept of biohacking, offering a clear and concise definition that sets the stage for the exploration that follows.

Biohacking is a dynamic practice rooted in the idea that our bodies are not set in stone. Instead, they are adaptable systems, responsive to various inputs and manipulations. It's the realization that our well-being is not solely dictated by genetics or fate but can be influenced and improved through our conscious efforts.

At its core, biohacking is a blend of self-experimentation and data-driven methods. It's about taking an active role in your own health and well-being, akin to a scientist conducting experiments in a lab. It's about collecting data, analyzing results, and making informed decisions based on evidence.

Biohackers understand that there is no one-size-fits-all solution. What works for one person may not work for another. Therefore, they embrace the idea of personalized optimization. It's about finding the unique strategies and interventions that work best for your body and lifestyle.

In the chapters that follow, we'll delve deeper into the principles and practices of biohacking, exploring how you can apply these concepts to unlock your full potential, achieve better health, and elevate your performance to new heights. But before we embark on this journey, let's solidify our understanding of the core concept: biohacking is the art of optimizing one's health and performance through self-experimentation and data-driven methods. It's a path to empowerment, where you become the master of your own biology.

The Growing Popularity of Biohacking

The world of biohacking is not confined to the fringes of scientific research or the domain of a select few. In recent years, there has been a notable surge in interest and engagement with biohacking practices among the general population. This chapter delves into the factors driving this growing popularity and examines the widespread curiosity surrounding biohacking.

The rise of the internet and social media has played a significant role in disseminating information about biohacking. Online communities, forums, and platforms have allowed biohackers to share their experiences, experiments, and success stories. As information spreads, more individuals are exposed to the concept and possibilities of biohacking, leading to increased curiosity and engagement.

Another driving force behind the popularity of biohacking is the desire for self-improvement and personal growth. In a fast-paced world where stress, sedentary lifestyles, and health concerns abound, people are increasingly seeking ways to optimize their physical and mental well-being. Biohacking offers a proactive approach to achieving these goals, resonating with individuals looking to take control of their health and performance.

Celebrities and influential figures have also contributed to the rise of biohacking in popular culture. When high-profile individuals openly discuss their biohacking experiences and the benefits they've derived, it tends to pique the curiosity of their followers and fans. The endorsement of biohacking practices by well-known personalities further propels the movement into the mainstream.

Moreover, advancements in technology have made biohacking more accessible than ever before. Wearable devices, health-tracking apps, and affordable genetic testing kits have empowered individuals to monitor and modify various aspects of their health. This democratization of biohacking tools has removed barriers and made self-improvement more achievable for a broader audience.

As we explore the growing popularity of biohacking, it becomes evident that this movement is not limited to a niche community but has found its way into the hearts and minds of people from all walks of life. It represents a shift towards proactive health management and personal optimization—a shift that is likely to continue evolving in the years to come. In the chapters ahead, we will delve deeper into the core principles and practices of biohacking, enabling you to harness the power of self-experimentation and data-driven methods for your own benefit.

The Human Body as a Complex System

In the world of biohacking, the human body is not merely a sum of its parts but a remarkably intricate and interconnected system. To embark on a journey of biohacking is to embrace this fundamental truth. This chapter peels back the layers of complexity that shroud our physiology, setting the stage for the principles and practices that underpin biohacking.

Our bodies are a tapestry of interwoven systems, each playing a vital role in maintaining equilibrium. From the cardiovascular system, which transports oxygen and nutrients, to the endocrine system, which regulates hormones and metabolism, these systems function harmoniously to sustain life. It is this intricate symphony of systems that allows us to adapt to changing environments and challenges.

A central tenet of biohacking is recognizing that these systems are not isolated; they are interconnected, influencing one another in a delicate dance. When we intervene in one area, we send ripples throughout the entire system. This interconnectedness is exemplified by the profound impact of exercise on not only our muscles but also our cardiovascular, endocrine, and nervous systems.

Understanding this complexity is essential for biohackers. It forms the bedrock upon which all biohacking principles rest. When you engage in self-experimentation, whether it's altering your diet, sleep patterns, or exercise routines, you are navigating the intricate web of these bodily systems. It's akin to being a conductor leading an orchestra, making adjustments to achieve the perfect harmony.

The body's remarkable ability to adapt is both a blessing and a challenge for biohackers. It means that changes, whether positive or negative, can reverberate throughout the system. It underscores the importance of precise experimentation and data-driven decision-making. Biohackers must learn to read the body's responses and fine-tune their interventions accordingly.

In essence, biohacking is about mastering this complexity, uncovering the unique symphony that is your own physiology, and learning to play the notes that lead to optimal health and performance. As we delve deeper into the principles of biohacking in the chapters that follow, remember this foundational truth: your body is a complex system, and biohacking is the art of orchestrating it to achieve your desired outcomes.

Systems Thinking in Biohacking

Biohacking, at its core, is not a reductionist endeavor but a holistic exploration of the human body's intricacies. It's an approach that recognizes the interplay between various bodily systems and understands that health and performance are the products of this dynamic orchestration. In this chapter, we delve into the critical concept of systems thinking in biohacking and how it shapes the way we optimize our biology.

Our bodies are not composed of isolated components that operate independently. Instead, they function as an integrated whole, where each system influences and is influenced by the others. For instance, the state of your cardiovascular system can impact your energy levels, cognitive function, and even your emotional well-being.

Systems thinking in biohacking entails examining the bigger picture, understanding how different systems interact, and appreciating the ripple effect that changes in one area can have throughout the body. This approach challenges the notion of addressing symptoms in isolation and encourages a more comprehensive understanding of health and performance.

When biohackers make interventions in their lives, such as altering their diets, optimizing sleep, or modifying exercise routines, they do so with an awareness of how these changes may affect multiple systems. For example, a change in diet can influence not only weight but also energy levels, hormone balance, and mental clarity. Biohackers recognize these interdependencies and aim to create interventions that yield positive outcomes across multiple fronts.

Furthermore, biohacking embraces the idea that no single system operates in isolation; they are all connected. The nervous system communicates with the endocrine system, which, in turn, impacts the immune system. This interconnectedness means that biohacking interventions should be designed to optimize the entire ecosystem of the body, rather than just isolated components.

In essence, systems thinking in biohacking represents a paradigm shift in how we approach health and performance. It requires us to view the body as a symphony of systems, where harmony and balance lead to optimal outcomes. As we proceed through the chapters of this book, you'll discover how biohackers apply systems thinking to create personalized strategies that improve overall well-being and push the boundaries of human potential.

The Importance of Homeostasis

In the world of biohacking, the concept of homeostasis stands as a guiding principle. It acknowledges that the human body is not a static entity but a dynamic, self-regulating system that constantly strives to maintain balance. This chapter highlights the vital role of homeostasis and how biohacking seeks to optimize this delicate equilibrium.

Homeostasis is the body's innate ability to maintain stable conditions within a narrow range, despite external influences. It ensures that our temperature, blood pressure, pH levels, and countless other parameters remain within the optimal range for cellular function. It's the body's way of ensuring that we can adapt and thrive in a constantly changing world.

Biohackers recognize that homeostasis is not a static state but a dynamic process. It is the body's response to the ever-shifting demands placed upon it. When we subject our bodies to stress, whether physical, mental, or environmental, it triggers a cascade of responses aimed at restoring equilibrium.

The practice of biohacking leverages this principle by intentionally subjecting the body to controlled stressors. For instance, through targeted exercise routines, biohackers push their physical limits, challenging muscles, cardiovascular systems, and even hormonal responses. By doing so, they provoke the body to adapt and improve its performance in response to these stressors.

Nutrition also plays a significant role in optimizing homeostasis. Biohackers understand that what we eat can either support or disrupt the body's delicate balance. Therefore, they tailor their diets to provide the nutrients and energy needed for optimal function while minimizing the disruptions that can result from poor dietary choices.

Additionally, biohackers appreciate that sleep, stress management, and other lifestyle factors are essential for maintaining homeostasis. Sleep, for example, is a critical time when the body repairs, regenerates, and restores balance. Biohackers prioritize sleep optimization to ensure their bodies can effectively maintain homeostasis.

In essence, biohacking seeks to optimize homeostasis by intelligently challenging and supporting the body's natural tendency to maintain balance. It's a practice that leverages the body's remarkable adaptability to promote not only survival but also thriving. As we continue our journey through the principles and practices of biohacking, keep in mind the central role that homeostasis plays in achieving optimal health and performance.

Self-Experimentation

Biohacking is inherently a science, and at its core lies the practice of self-experimentation. It's a deliberate and systematic approach to understanding how specific interventions impact one's health and performance. In this chapter, we delve into the art and science of self-experimentation and how it serves as the cornerstone of biohacking.

Self-experimentation begins with curiosity—a burning desire to understand one's own body and how it responds to various stimuli. Biohackers are like investigators, seeking answers to questions that revolve around health, vitality, and peak performance. What happens when I tweak my diet? How does my body react to different sleep patterns? What exercise regimen yields the best results? These are the questions that fuel the biohacker's curiosity.

The process of self-experimentation is systematic and data-driven. It involves setting clear hypotheses, designing controlled experiments, and meticulously tracking data. For example, a biohacker interested in optimizing their sleep might experiment with different sleep schedules, monitor sleep quality using wearables, and record daily observations in a journal.

Crucially, self-experimentation requires objectivity. Biohackers are not bound by preconceived notions or assumptions. They approach their experiments with an open mind, acknowledging that their initial hypotheses may be proven wrong. They embrace the scientific method, using evidence to guide their decisions and conclusions.

Moreover, self-experimentation is iterative. Biohackers understand that the body is a dynamic system, and what works today may not work tomorrow. As such, they are willing to adapt and refine their approaches based on the data they gather and the feedback their bodies provide.

Ethical considerations are paramount in self-experimentation. Biohackers prioritize safety and responsible experimentation. They understand that pushing the boundaries of knowledge should not come at the expense of their well-being. Therefore, they take measures to minimize risks, seek professional guidance when necessary, and prioritize ethical and responsible practices.

The biohacker's journey of self-experimentation is a continuous and evolving process. It's an exploration of the body's potential, an ongoing quest for optimal health and performance. As we navigate through the principles and practices of biohacking in the chapters ahead, remember that self-experimentation is the driving force behind this journey—an empowering process that enables you to unlock the secrets of your own biology.

Data Collection and Analysis

In the world of biohacking, data reigns supreme. It is the compass that guides biohackers on their journey to optimizing health and performance. This chapter explores the pivotal role of data in biohacking, covering the collection, analysis, and interpretation of a wide range of metrics and biomarkers.

Data collection in biohacking is akin to assembling puzzle pieces to create a comprehensive picture of one's health and well-being. Biohackers meticulously gather data on various aspects of their lives, including sleep patterns, nutrition, exercise routines, and physiological biomarkers. The goal is to create a detailed map of how different interventions and lifestyle choices impact the body.

Sleep tracking is a prominent aspect of data collection. Biohackers use wearables and apps to monitor the duration and quality of their sleep. This data helps them identify patterns, disruptions, and areas for improvement in their sleep hygiene.

Nutrition data plays a critical role in optimizing dietary choices. Biohackers may track macronutrient intake, micronutrient levels, and even specific dietary protocols to assess their impact on energy levels, mood, and overall health.

Exercise data includes tracking workout routines, monitoring heart rate variability, and recording fitness progress. This information helps biohackers fine-tune their exercise regimens to achieve specific goals, whether it's building muscle, improving endurance, or enhancing overall fitness.

Physiological biomarkers are the gold standard in data-driven biohacking. Blood tests, hormone panels, genetic analyses, and other biomarker assessments provide concrete data on internal health. These markers allow biohackers to detect deficiencies, imbalances, or potential health risks and make targeted interventions.

Data analysis is the next crucial step. Biohackers don't merely collect data; they derive insights from it. They look for patterns, correlations, and cause-and-effect relationships. For instance, they may discover that a particular dietary change leads to improved sleep quality or that specific supplements influence biomarker levels.

Interpreting data requires a scientific mindset. Biohackers rely on critical thinking and evidence-based reasoning to draw conclusions. They recognize that correlation does not imply causation and strive for objectivity in their analysis.

Furthermore, data collection and analysis are ongoing processes in biohacking. Biohackers continuously gather new data, compare results, and refine their interventions based on their findings. It's a journey of self-discovery guided by objective information.

In essence, data collection and analysis are the backbone of biohacking, providing the insights and evidence needed to make informed decisions about health and performance optimization. As we delve into the practical applications of biohacking in the chapters ahead, remember that data is your ally—a valuable tool that empowers you to take control of your biology and achieve your goals.

The Role of Technology in Biohacking

Technology has ushered in a new era of biohacking, making the practice more accessible, precise, and data-driven than ever before. This chapter shines a spotlight on the critical role that technology plays in biohacking, particularly in data collection and analysis, through the use of wearables, apps, and digital tools.

Wearables have revolutionized how biohackers monitor and collect data on their bodies. Devices such as smartwatches, fitness trackers, and health monitors have become indispensable tools in the biohacker's arsenal. They provide real-time information on various health metrics, including heart rate, sleep patterns, physical activity, and even stress levels.

Sleep tracking wearables, for instance, offer insights into sleep duration, sleep stages, and disturbances throughout the night. Biohackers use this data to optimize their sleep hygiene and routines.

Nutrition apps and trackers allow biohackers to log their dietary intake, track macronutrients, and even scan barcodes for nutritional information. This information helps biohackers make informed choices about their diets and identify patterns that may impact their health and performance.

Exercise enthusiasts benefit from fitness trackers that monitor heart rate, calories burned, and exercise intensity. These wearables assist biohackers in tailoring their workout routines to achieve specific fitness goals.

Moreover, technology enables biohackers to quantify and analyze physiological biomarkers with precision. Blood glucose monitors, continuous glucose monitors (CGMs), genetic testing kits, and at-home diagnostic devices provide invaluable data for health optimization. Biohackers can assess the impact of dietary changes, supplements, or lifestyle interventions on these biomarkers, leading to evidence-based decisions.

Data integration platforms and biohacking apps allow biohackers to aggregate data from various sources, providing a comprehensive view of their health and performance. These platforms often employ artificial intelligence and machine learning algorithms to identify trends, anomalies, and opportunities for improvement.

While technology empowers biohackers with data, it's crucial to emphasize responsible and secure data management. Biohackers prioritize data privacy and security, understanding the sensitivity of the information they collect.

The role of technology in biohacking is not limited to data collection alone; it extends to data analysis, interpretation, and visualization. Biohackers leverage digital tools to extract actionable insights from the vast troves of data they accumulate.

In essence, technology is the enabler that propels biohacking into the digital age. It equips biohackers with the tools they need to gather, analyze, and harness data to optimize their health and performance. As we navigate through the practical applications of biohacking in the upcoming chapters, remember that technology is your ally in this journey—a partner that empowers you to unlock the potential of your biology.

Pioneers of Biohacking - Their Journeys and Achievements

In the world of biohacking, there exist exceptional individuals whose journeys and achievements have left an indelible mark on the landscape of self-improvement. In this chapter, we turn our attention to these trailblazers and their remarkable experiences and accomplishments.

Dave Asprey: The Bulletproof Innovator

Dave Asprey embarked on a journey fueled by a desire to enhance cognitive performance and vitality. His creation of Bulletproof Coffee, a blend of high-quality coffee, grass-fed butter, and MCT oil, gained worldwide attention for its potential to boost mental clarity and energy. Asprey's unwavering commitment to optimal nutrition and lifestyle practices led to the development of the Bulletproof Diet, which prioritizes low-toxin, high-nutrient foods. His pioneering spirit has inspired countless individuals to take charge of their health and well-being through biohacking.

Ben Greenfield: Pushing the Boundaries of Human Performance

Ben Greenfield's journey is characterized by his relentless pursuit of cutting-edge fitness, nutrition, and recovery strategies. As an elite athlete, coach, and author, he has continually pushed the boundaries of physical and mental capabilities. Greenfield's experimentation with techniques like cold exposure, sauna therapy, and personalized nutrition has not only elevated his own athletic prowess but has also paved the way for others to optimize their physical and mental performance. His emphasis on data-driven self-experimentation has empowered countless individuals to achieve their fitness and health goals.

Rhonda Patrick: Bridging Nutrition and Longevity

Dr. Rhonda Patrick's journey is deeply rooted in scientific inquiry and a dedication to unraveling the intricate connections between nutrition, genetics, and longevity. Her groundbreaking research into the role of micronutrients, such as vitamin D and sulforaphane, in cellular health has illuminated practical interventions for optimizing well-being. Dr. Patrick's ability to translate complex scientific concepts into actionable insights through her podcast and online presence has contributed to greater awareness and informed decision-making in the realms of health and longevity.

Tim Ferriss: Deconstructing Excellence and Human Potential

Tim Ferriss, a prolific author, entrepreneur, and biohacker, embarked on a mission to deconstruct excellence and uncover the secrets of human potential. Through his influential book "The 4-Hour Body," Ferriss shared his experiments with unconventional techniques, ranging from rapid fat loss to muscle gain. His practical and data-driven approach to self-improvement has resonated with millions, motivating them to adopt innovative strategies for enhancing various aspects of their lives.

David Sinclair: Pioneering Anti-Aging Research

Dr. David Sinclair's journey as a biologist and geneticist has been marked by groundbreaking discoveries in the field of aging and longevity. His pioneering work on molecules like NAD+ and resveratrol has expanded our understanding of cellular aging and potential interventions. Dr. Sinclair's dedication to unraveling the mysteries of aging holds the promise of revolutionizing our approach to healthspan and lifespan extension.

Elizabeth Parrish: A Bold Leap into Genetic Interventions

Elizabeth Parrish's journey is characterized by her audacious decision to become one of the first individuals to undergo gene therapy for aging. As the CEO of BioViva, she advocates for genetic interventions aimed at extending healthspan. Parrish's pioneering spirit exemplifies the potential of genetic advancements in the quest for longevity.

Josiah Zayner: A Trailblazer in Democratizing Biotechnology

Josiah Zayner's journey reflects a fervent passion for democratizing biotechnology and self-experimentation. A former NASA scientist, Zayner garnered attention for self-administering gene-editing treatments. He has been a tireless advocate for individual empowerment in the realm of scientific exploration, challenging traditional norms and inspiring discussions about the role of biohackers in pushing the boundaries of scientific discovery.

Natasha Vita-More: Bridging Art, Science, and Philosophy

Natasha Vita-More's journey is a testament to her ability to bridge the realms of art, science, and philosophy in the context of human enhancement. Her pioneering work in cryonics and life extension explores the intersection of aesthetics and the pursuit of longevity. Vita-More's creative and philosophical contributions inspire deep contemplation on the ethical and existential dimensions of biohacking.

Andrew Huberman: Unraveling the Mysteries of the Brain

Dr. Andrew Huberman's journey as a neuroscientist has focused on unraveling the science of stress, sleep, and vision. His research has provided valuable insights into optimizing brain function and overall well-being. Huberman's dedication to understanding the complexities of the human brain has paved the way for strategies to enhance cognitive health and performance.

Max Lugavere: Championing Brain Health

Max Lugavere's journey is centered around the critical importance of brain health and cognitive optimization. His work in the field of nutrition and neurology has empowered individuals to prioritize brain health as a cornerstone of overall well-being. Lugavere's advocacy for evidence-based practices underscores the significance of informed choices in the pursuit of cognitive enhancement.

These remarkable biohackers serve as beacons of inspiration for those embarking on their own journeys of self-improvement. As we delve into the practical applications of biohacking in the upcoming chapters, let us remember that while these individuals have achieved remarkable results, biohacking is ultimately a deeply personal journey, and each biohacker's achievements are a testament to the boundless potential of human optimization.

100 Biohacks for Optimal Health and Wellness

In this comprehensive section, we delve into 100 innovative biohacks that cater to a wide range of goals - from enhancing physical fitness and mental clarity to achieving longevity and emotional wellbeing. Biohacking, at its core, is about making small, incremental lifestyle changes that make a significant impact on your overall quality of life. It's about understanding your body and mind in profound ways and using this knowledge to optimize your health.

These 100 biohacks are designed for everyone, whether you're a beginner curious about simple lifestyle tweaks or a seasoned biohacker looking for advanced techniques. We'll explore methods that range from nutritional adjustments, such as intermittent fasting and ketogenic diets, to high-tech interventions like genetic editing and neurofeedback.

Each hack is rooted in the principle of self-experimentation and personalization. The idea is to empower you to take control of your own health by providing a toolkit of diverse options. You'll find strategies to enhance your physical endurance, cognitive capabilities, and emotional resilience, alongside techniques to balance your internal systems for optimal performance.

Remember, biohacking is as much about the journey as it is about the destination. It's an ongoing process of exploration, learning, and adaptation. As you embark on this journey, keep an open mind, listen to your body, and be ready to embrace the transformative power of biohacking. Let's unlock your full potential with these 100 biohacks!

Intermittent Fasting: Experiment with fasting intervals to enhance metabolism.

Intermittent fasting has rapidly gained popularity as a potent method to enhance metabolism and overall health. This approach alternates between periods of fasting and eating, challenging traditional beliefs about daily meal frequency. Its effectiveness lies in the physiological changes that occur during fasting: the body shifts from using glucose for energy to tapping into stored fat, a process that can lead to weight loss and improved metabolic health. Dr. Jason Fung, a leading expert in intermittent fasting, states, "Intermittent fasting is a powerful approach to eating that is becoming very popular because it can help you lose weight while feeling great" (Fung, 2016). Fung emphasizes that intermittent fasting is more about when you eat rather than what you eat.

Fasting intervals can vary, with the 16/8 method being one of the most common, where you fast for 16 hours and eat during an 8-hour window. Another approach is the 5:2 method, where you eat normally for five days of the week and significantly reduce calorie intake for the other two. Dr. Mark Mattson, a neuroscientist at the National Institute on Aging, advocates for the neuroprotective benefits of intermittent fasting, noting, "Fasting has the potential to delay aging and help prevent and treat diseases while minimizing the side effects caused by chronic dietary interventions" (Mattson, 2014). This approach not only aids in weight management but also improves insulin sensitivity, lowers the risk of type 2 diabetes, and enhances brain health.

Intermittent fasting represents a paradigm shift in dietary habits, moving away from the traditional three-meals-a-day structure. It's a flexible approach, adaptable to different lifestyles and dietary needs, making it a practical option for many seeking to improve their health through biohacking.

Cold Showers: Use cold exposure to improve circulation and resilience.

Cold showers, a cornerstone practice in the biohacking community, leverage the power of cold exposure to improve circulation and resilience. This practice involves deliberately exposing oneself to cold water, which triggers a range of physiological responses beneficial to health. One of the primary effects is the improvement of blood circulation, as cold water causes blood vessels to constrict and then dilate, enhancing blood flow. Wim Hof, known for his cold endurance feats, advocates for cold showers, stating, "A cold shower a day keeps the doctor away" (Hof, 2019). Hof emphasizes the benefits of improved circulation and immune response from regular cold exposure.

Besides circulation, cold showers are renowned for their ability to enhance mental resilience. The initial shock of cold water requires a level of mental fortitude and acclimatization. Over time, this practice strengthens not only the body's response to stress but also the mind's. Dr. Rhonda Patrick, a biomedical scientist, notes, "Cold exposure, such as cold showers, can increase norepinephrine up to five-fold in the brain, which can help with focus and attention" (Patrick, 2017). This increase in norepinephrine, a key neurotransmitter and hormone, not only improves focus but also contributes to mood elevation.

Integrating cold showers into daily routines is a simple yet profound biohack. Starting with just a few seconds and gradually increasing the duration makes the practice more adaptable. This method, while initially uncomfortable, offers long-term benefits, including enhanced immune function, improved skin and hair health, and increased energy levels. Cold showers symbolize a direct, no-frills approach to improving physical and mental health.

High-Intensity Interval Training (HIIT): Boost fitness efficiently.

High-Intensity Interval Training (HIIT) stands as a highly efficient method to boost fitness, compressing intense physical exertion into short timeframes. This approach alternates short bursts of intense exercise with periods of rest or lower-intensity activity. The effectiveness of HIIT lies in its ability to provide significant fitness gains within a reduced duration compared to traditional, longer-duration exercise routines. "HIIT can provide similar or greater benefits for health and fitness than moderate-intensity continuous training," states Dr. Martin Gibala, a professor of kinesiology at McMaster University (Gibala, 2017). Gibala's research highlights HIIT's capacity to improve aerobic fitness, cardiovascular health, and insulin sensitivity.

A typical HIIT session may last from 15 to 30 minutes, with exercises varying from sprinting and cycling to bodyweight movements. The key component is the intensity; during the high-intensity phases, effort levels should be close to maximum. "High-intensity interval training is a time-efficient strategy to get the benefits typically associated with longer bouts of traditional cardio," confirms Dr. Tabata, a Japanese researcher whose studies on interval training have been foundational (Tabata, 1996). His protocol, known as the Tabata method, involves 20 seconds of ultra-intense exercise followed by 10 seconds of rest, repeated for 4 minutes.

The appeal of HIIT lies in its adaptability to various fitness levels and settings, requiring minimal equipment. It's known for burning a high number of calories in a short period and creating a metabolic disturbance that can lead to increased fat burning long after the workout has ended. This post-exercise period, often referred to as the 'afterburn effect' or excess post-exercise oxygen consumption (EPOC), is a key element in HIIT's effectiveness for weight loss and metabolic health.

Meditation: Enhance mental clarity and stress management.

Meditation, a core practice in both ancient traditions and modern biohacking, enhances mental clarity and manages stress. This practice involves focusing the mind and training attention, leading to a state of mental calm and clarity. Regular meditation has been linked to reduced levels of stress and anxiety, along with improved cognitive function and emotional well-being. Neuroscientist Dr. Sara Lazar's research at Harvard University demonstrates that meditation can actually change the structure of the brain, enhancing areas responsible for attention and emotional regulation (Lazar, 2005). Lazar's findings underline meditation's potential to profoundly impact mental health.

Stress reduction is one of the most well-known benefits of meditation. By promoting relaxation and a sense of peace, meditation can lower cortisol levels, the body's primary stress hormone. Jon Kabat-Zinn, the founder of the Mindfulness-Based Stress Reduction program, asserts, "The awareness that arises from paying attention, on purpose, in the present moment, and non-judgmentally, has the potential to transform our relationship to our problems and to our lives" (Kabat-Zinn, 1990). His work emphasizes meditation's role in altering one's perception of stress and challenges.

Meditation practices vary widely, from mindfulness, which involves observing thoughts and sensations without judgment, to concentration meditations, which focus on a single point of reference. The practice is accessible to everyone, requiring no special equipment or environment. Its versatility and effectiveness make meditation a favored biohack for improving mental health, offering a straightforward approach to enhancing life quality through mental training.

Sleep Tracking: Use technology to analyze and improve sleep quality.

Sleep tracking, a pivotal biohacking tool, leverages technology to analyze and improve sleep quality. This approach uses devices such as smartwatches, fitness trackers, or smartphone apps to monitor various aspects of sleep, including duration, stages (like REM and deep sleep), and disturbances. The data gathered provides insights into sleep patterns, helping to identify areas for improvement. Dr. Matthew Walker, a professor of neuroscience and psychology and the author of "Why We Sleep," emphasizes the importance of understanding sleep patterns: "By tracking our sleep, we can make informed decisions about habits and behaviors that are beneficial or detrimental to sleep health" (Walker, 2017). This information is crucial in a society where sleep deprivation is increasingly common.

The use of sleep tracking technologies has grown exponentially, offering users detailed feedback on their sleep. These devices often track movements and heart rate to estimate sleep stages, providing a comprehensive overview of sleep quality. "Sleep trackers can provide valuable data about your rest patterns and rhythms," states Dr. Rebecca Robbins, a postdoctoral researcher at Brigham and Women's Hospital and Harvard Medical School (Robbins, 2019). This data can lead to actionable insights, such as adjusting bedtime routines, sleep environment, or daily habits to enhance sleep quality.

Effective sleep tracking goes beyond merely quantifying hours slept; it delves into the quality of sleep and its impact on overall health. Understanding sleep patterns can lead to better management of stress, improved cognitive function, and better physical health. As a biohacking tool, sleep tracking stands out for its ability

Ketogenic Diet: Try a high-fat, low-carb diet for energy and weight loss.

The ketogenic diet, a significant shift in traditional dietary habits, emphasizes a high-fat, low-carbohydrate regimen to stimulate energy and weight loss. By drastically reducing carbohydrate intake and replacing it with fat, the body enters a metabolic state known as ketosis. In this state, the body becomes incredibly efficient at burning fat for energy. Dr. Eric Westman, a leading researcher in low-carbohydrate diets, states, "The keto diet is a very effective way of achieving weight loss, improving blood sugar control, and even improving markers of heart disease" (Westman, 2014). This approach challenges conventional dietary guidelines, offering an alternative path to those struggling with traditional diet plans.

The ketogenic diet involves a significant reduction in carbohydrate consumption, limiting it to about 20 to 50 grams per day, and replacing it with healthy fats and moderate protein. This shift away from carbs prevents spikes in blood sugar, leading to improved insulin sensitivity and reduced inflammation. "When you're in ketosis, your body burns fat more efficiently," explains Dr. Dominic D'Agostino, an associate professor at the University of South Florida and a researcher in metabolic therapies (D'Agostino, 2015). D'Agostino highlights ketosis as a state where the body uses fat, rather than glucose, as its primary energy source.

Apart from weight loss, the ketogenic diet is known for its potential therapeutic effects on various neurological disorders, including epilepsy and Alzheimer's disease. It has also gained popularity for its ability to increase energy levels and mental clarity. The ketogenic diet represents a radical departure from conventional high-carbohydrate diets, offering a biohacking tool for those seeking alternative methods for weight loss and health optimization.

Nootropics: Explore cognitive enhancers for brain function.

Nootropics, often referred to as 'smart drugs' or cognitive enhancers, are substances that can boost brain performance. They are becoming increasingly popular in the biohacking community for their potential to improve memory, focus, creativity, intelligence, and motivation. "Nootropics are substances that improve mental function while doing no harm," says Dr. Corneliu E. Giurgea, the psychologist and chemist who coined the term (Giurgea, 1972). His pioneering work laid the foundation for the modern fascination with these cognitive enhancers.

The range of nootropics includes both natural and synthetic compounds. Caffeine, one of the most widely consumed nootropics, is praised for its ability to enhance alertness and concentration. More complex nootropics, like racetams and modafinil, are believed to boost brain function by increasing neurotransmitter activity. "Modafinil seems to be the first 'smart drug' that is reasonably safe for healthy people," reported Dr. Barbara Sahakian, a professor at the University of Cambridge known for her research on cognitive enhancers (Sahakian, 2015). Her research suggests that modafinil in particular may improve decision-making and planning skills.

While nootropics offer promising benefits for cognitive enhancement, there is ongoing debate and research about their long-term effects and efficacy. They are part of a larger trend in biohacking that seeks to maximize human potential. As Dr. Giurgea's initial assertion about their safety and efficacy remains a guiding principle, ongoing research and individual experimentation continue to shape the world of nootropics.

Gratitude Journaling: Boost mental health and perspective.

Gratitude journaling, a simple yet profoundly effective biohack, has gained traction for its ability to enhance mental health and shift perspective. This practice involves regularly writing down things for which one is grateful, fostering a heightened sense of well-being and positivity. Psychologists Dr. Robert A. Emmons and Dr. Michael E. McCullough, leading researchers on gratitude, found significant mental health benefits from the practice of gratitude journaling. "Gratitude journaling leads to reduced depressive symptoms and increased happiness," Dr. Emmons explains (Emmons & McCullough, 2003). Their research underscores the power of gratitude in altering one's mental landscape.

The act of gratitude journaling shifts focus from negative or stressful aspects of life to positive ones, fostering a sense of contentment and reducing stress and anxiety. This practice doesn't just improve mood in the short term; it can lead to lasting increases in happiness. According to Dr. Martin Seligman, a pioneer in the field of positive psychology, "Writing about the things for which we are grateful can significantly increase well-being and life satisfaction" (Seligman, 2005). Seligman's work emphasizes the long-term benefits of cultivating gratitude.

Gratitude journaling is more than just a feel-good exercise; it's a tool that can reshape thinking patterns, leading to a more optimistic and resilient mindset. Its simplicity makes it accessible to anyone and can be seamlessly integrated into daily routines. As a biohacking technique, it stands out for its efficacy and ease of implementation, making it a valuable practice for those seeking to enhance their mental health and overall outlook on life.

Standing Desk: Reduce sedentary lifestyle impacts.

Standing desks have become a popular solution in the biohacking community to mitigate the negative impacts of a sedentary lifestyle. By allowing individuals to stand while working, these desks encourage more movement and less sitting, which is often associated with various health risks. Dr. James Levine, a professor of medicine at the Mayo Clinic, known for his research on sitting, notes, "The simple act of standing instead of sitting may significantly reduce your risk of heart disease, diabetes, and a host of other health issues" (Levine, 2015). His research highlights the importance of reducing sedentary time for overall health.

The transition to standing desks addresses the issue of prolonged sitting, which is linked to increased risks of obesity, heart disease, and diabetes, among other health concerns. "Sitting is more dangerous than smoking, kills more people than HIV, and is more treacherous than parachuting. We are sitting ourselves to death," says Dr. Levine (Levine, 2014). Standing desks not only promote better posture and reduce back pain but also have been shown to improve mood and energy levels.

Incorporating standing desks into daily routines represents a simple yet effective biohack to combat the sedentary habits of modern life. This shift in work environment encourages a more active lifestyle, aligning with the biohacking ethos of making small, sustainable changes for significant health benefits. The standing desk is a testament to the principle that sometimes, the simplest interventions can lead to the most profound health improvements.

Bulletproof Coffee: Start your day with coffee mixed with MCT oil and butter.

Bulletproof Coffee, a novel concoction in the biohacking community, combines coffee with MCT (Medium Chain Triglyceride) oil and unsalted butter, often from grass-fed cows. This blend is touted for its ability to provide sustained energy and improved cognitive function. The creator of Bulletproof Coffee, Dave Asprey, claims, "When you drink Bulletproof Coffee, you'll feel the difference with your first cup" (Asprey, 2014). Asprey promotes this drink as a tool for improved mental clarity and prolonged energy without the typical caffeine crash.

The concept behind Bulletproof Coffee is that the combination of caffeine with fats from MCT oil and butter slows the body's absorption of caffeine, providing a more sustained release of energy. MCT oil is known for its ability to be rapidly absorbed and metabolized by the body, providing a quick source of energy. Nutritionist Dr. Mary Newport highlights the benefits of MCT oil, stating, "MCTs are a unique form of fat that require less energy and enzymes to be digested" (Newport, 2015). This makes Bulletproof Coffee particularly appealing for those following a ketogenic diet, as it aligns with the diet's high-fat, low-carb approach.

Bulletproof Coffee has gained a following among biohackers and those seeking a morning boost without the hunger pangs often associated with a traditional coffee-only breakfast. This drink serves as more than just a caffeine kick; it's part of a lifestyle aimed at maximizing physical and cognitive performance.

Mindfulness Breathing Exercises: Enhance focus and calmness.

Mindfulness breathing exercises, a fundamental technique in the realm of biohacking, focus on controlled breathing to enhance mental focus and calmness. By consciously regulating breath, these exercises bring attention to the present moment, reducing stress and improving concentration. Dr. Herbert Benson, a pioneer in mind-body medicine, emphasizes the impact of controlled breathing on the body's stress response: "Breathing exercises can promote a relaxation response, counteracting the harmful effects of chronic stress" (Benson, 1975). Benson's research underscores the importance of such practices for mental and physical health.

These exercises typically involve deep, rhythmic breathing, sometimes with a specific pattern of inhalation, holding the breath, and exhalation. Dr. Andrew Weil, a leader in integrative medicine, advocates for the 4-7-8 breathing technique, stating, "This simple breathing exercise can be a powerful tool to reset your stress response and promote a sense of calm" (Weil, 2017). Weil's technique is just one example of how structured breathing can be used to manage stress and anxiety.

Incorporating mindfulness breathing exercises into daily routines can lead to significant improvements in mental clarity, emotional stability, and overall well-being. This practice is not only beneficial for those facing high stress or anxiety but is also valuable for anyone looking to enhance their cognitive function and maintain a calm, focused state of mind. As a biohack, mindfulness breathing is accessible, requires no special equipment, and can be practiced anywhere, making it a versatile tool for enhancing mental health.

Wearable Fitness Trackers: Monitor physical activity and health metrics.

Wearable fitness trackers have revolutionized the way individuals monitor their physical activity and health metrics, becoming a staple in the biohacking community. These devices track a range of data, including steps taken, calories burned, heart rate, and sleep patterns. Dr. Michael Snyder, a leader in the field of genomics and wearables, points out, "Wearable devices provide a continuous stream of health and fitness data, offering unprecedented insights into our daily lives" (Snyder, 2018). Snyder's research emphasizes the potential of wearables in personal health monitoring and disease prevention.

These trackers encourage users to be more active and make healthier choices by providing real-time feedback and setting achievable goals. The data collected can reveal patterns and trends in physical activity, sleep, and even stress levels, helping users to make informed decisions about their health. "Wearables are not just fitness trackers; they are wellness tools. They can guide users towards healthier habits and early detection of health issues," states Dr. Gregory Marcus, a cardiologist specializing in the use of wearables for heart health (Marcus, 2019).

Incorporating wearable fitness trackers into a daily routine is a practical biohack for anyone looking to improve their physical health. These devices serve as a constant reminder and motivator, encouraging increased physical activity and awareness of health metrics. The integration of wearables into health and fitness regimes represents a shift towards more data-driven, personalized approaches to health optimization.

Blue Light Blocking Glasses: Reduce digital eye strain and improve sleep.

Blue light blocking glasses have become an essential tool in the biohacking toolkit, particularly for those looking to reduce digital eye strain and improve sleep quality in our screen-saturated world. These glasses are designed to filter out blue light emitted by screens, which can disrupt circadian rhythms and interfere with sleep. Dr. Charles Czeisler, a professor of sleep medicine at Harvard University, notes, "Exposure to blue light at night, emitted by electronics and energy-efficient lightbulbs, can disrupt our internal clock and adversely affect sleep" (Czeisler,

2013). His research underscores the impact of blue light on our natural sleep patterns.

The use of blue light blocking glasses is especially relevant in the evening when exposure to blue light can hinder the production of melatonin, the hormone responsible for regulating sleep-wake cycles. By filtering out blue light, these glasses can help maintain a natural circadian rhythm, leading to improved sleep quality and overall well-being. Dr. Harneet Walia, a doctor at the Cleveland Clinic's Sleep Disorders Center, supports this, stating, "Wearing blue light blocking glasses can improve sleep quality, especially for those who have high screen time exposure in the evening" (Walia, 2016).

Adopting blue light blocking glasses as part of a nightly routine is a simple yet effective biohack for those who spend significant time in front of screens, whether for work or leisure. This practice is a proactive step towards safeguarding one's circadian rhythm, enhancing sleep quality, and reducing the risk of digital eye strain.

DNA Testing: Personalize diet and exercise based on genetics.

DNA testing, increasingly popular in the realm of biohacking, offers a personalized approach to optimizing diet and exercise based on genetic makeup. By analyzing an individual's DNA, these tests can provide insights into how one's body might respond to different types of food and exercise, tailoring wellness strategies to each person's unique genetic profile. Dr. Ruth DeBusk, a dietitian and geneticist, explains, "Nutrigenomics—the relationship between nutrition and your genes—can influence how your body responds to different dietary choices" (DeBusk,

2004). This emerging field underscores the potential of genetic information in personalizing health strategies.

The information garnered from DNA tests can guide choices in nutritional plans, identifying potential food sensitivities, metabolic issues, and optimal nutrient types. Similarly, these tests can inform exercise regimens by identifying genetic factors related to muscle composition, endurance, and recovery. "Genetic testing in the realm of fitness can help identify the types of exercise that are most effective for an individual," states Dr. Robert Superko, a pioneer in the field of cardiogenomics (Superko, 2016).

Adopting DNA-based recommendations for diet and exercise is a biohacking strategy that goes beyond one-size-fits-all solutions. It offers a tailored approach, aligning lifestyle choices with an individual's genetic predispositions for optimal health and performance. As our understanding of the human genome evolves, DNA testing for personalized wellness plans represents a significant advancement in the pursuit of individualized health optimization.

Red Light Therapy: For skin health and circadian rhythm regulation.

Red Light Therapy, a biohacking method increasingly acknowledged for its benefits in skin health and circadian rhythm regulation, employs low-level wavelengths of red light to treat skin issues and improve overall well-being. This non-invasive therapy is known for its efficacy in promoting wound healing, reducing inflammation, and improving skin complexion. Dr. Michael Hamblin, an associate professor at Harvard Medical School and a leading expert on photomedicine, elaborates, "Red light therapy has been shown to promote mitochondrial function and increase ATP production, leading to rejuvenation of skin and muscle tissue" (Hamblin, 2016). His research indicates the potential of red light in cellular regeneration and repair.

Beyond skin health, red light therapy plays a role in regulating the body's circadian rhythm, which is crucial for overall health. Exposure to red light, particularly in the morning, can help reset the body's internal clock, enhancing sleep quality and mood. Dr. Hamblin adds, "Red light in the morning can synchronize your circadian rhythm, making it easier to wake up and feel energized" (Hamblin, 2017). This synchronization is especially beneficial in our modern lifestyle, where natural light exposure is often limited.

Incorporating red light therapy into daily routines has become a practical and effective biohack for those seeking non-pharmaceutical approaches to improve skin health and regulate sleep patterns. Its growing popularity is testament to its efficacy and ease of use, marking it as a valuable tool in the biohacker's arsenal for health optimization.

Yoga: Improve flexibility, balance, and mental well-being.

Yoga, a time-honored practice now embraced in the biohacking community, offers a holistic approach to improving flexibility, balance, and mental well-being. Rooted in ancient traditions, yoga combines physical postures, breathing exercises, and meditation to enhance overall health. Its benefits extend beyond physical fitness, encompassing mental and emotional health. Dr. Timothy

McCall, a physician and yoga therapist, states, "Yoga can lower stress, improve flexibility, enhance concentration, and contribute to a better overall quality of life" (McCall, 2007). His assertion highlights the multifaceted benefits of yoga in promoting holistic health.

Regular yoga practice is known to improve muscle tone, flexibility, and balance, reducing the risk of injury in daily life and other physical activities. Beyond the physical, yoga is acclaimed for its ability to calm the mind, reduce stress and anxiety, and enhance mindfulness. B.K.S. Iyengar, a renowned yoga teacher, notes, "Yoga helps you in maintaining balance in life, relationships, and within yourself" (Iyengar, 2005). Iyengar emphasizes yoga's role in fostering internal equilibrium and mental clarity.

As a biohack, yoga offers a low-impact, accessible way to enhance physical health while simultaneously nurturing mental and emotional resilience. Its adaptability to various skill levels and styles makes it a viable option for anyone seeking a comprehensive approach to health improvement. Yoga's integration of physical postures with mindful breathing and meditation creates a unique space for holistic self-care and wellness.

Polyphasic Sleep: Experiment with multiple short sleep periods.

Polyphasic sleep, a sleep pattern that involves multiple short sleep periods throughout the day, has gained attention in the biohacking community for its potential to maximize wakefulness and productivity. This unconventional sleep schedule breaks away from the traditional monophasic sleep cycle, aiming to reduce total sleep time while maintaining or even enhancing alertness and cognitive function. Dr. Claudio Stampi, a pioneer in polyphasic sleep research, advocates this method for certain situations, stating, "Polyphasic sleep strategies can improve prolonged sustained performance under conditions of sleep reduction" (Stampi, 1992). His research highlights the potential of polyphasic sleep in optimizing time and efficiency.

Common polyphasic sleep schedules include the Uberman, Everyman, and Dymaxion patterns, each consisting of a different number of naps and varying lengths of core sleep. Advocates of polyphasic sleep, like Steve Pavlina, a personal development coach who experimented with the Uberman schedule, claim significant increases in productivity and free time. "Polyphasic sleep can free up several hours a day, as your total sleep requirement decreases," says Pavlina (Pavlina, 2005).

While the idea of gaining extra waking hours is appealing, transitioning to a polyphasic sleep schedule requires careful planning and adaptation. It's important to note that polyphasic sleep may not be suitable for everyone, and long-term effects on health are still a subject of research. For those in the biohacking community seeking to push the boundaries of conventional sleep patterns, polyphasic sleep offers an intriguing possibility to reclaim hours and potentially enhance efficiency and productivity.

Heart Rate Variability Monitoring: Assess stress and recovery states.

Heart Rate Variability (HRV) monitoring, a key biohacking tool, assesses an individual's stress levels and recovery states by measuring the time variation between heartbeats. Unlike basic heart rate measurements, HRV offers deeper insights into the autonomic nervous system's function, reflecting the balance between the sympathetic (stress) and parasympathetic (rest) responses. Dr. Richard Gevirtz, a renowned researcher in HRV biofeedback, explains, "HRV is a significant indicator of physiological resilience and behavioral flexibility, reflecting an individual's capacity to adapt effectively to stress and environmental demands" (Gevirtz, 2015). His research underscores HRV's role as a critical marker of overall health and stress management.

By tracking HRV, individuals can gauge their body's response to stressors and their recovery status, making it a valuable tool for athletes, individuals with high-stress lifestyles, or those engaged in recovery from health issues. "Monitoring HRV can help people recognize the early signs of stress and take proactive steps to manage it," states Dr. Andrew Ahn, a cardiologist specializing in heart rhythm disorders (Ahn, 2018).

Incorporating HRV monitoring into a daily routine allows for a personalized approach to health and wellness, enabling individuals to tailor their activities, such as exercise, meditation, and sleep, based on their body's current needs. This practice exemplifies the biohacking ethos of using data to optimize health, providing a powerful lens through which to view and manage one's physiological state.

Supplement Stacking: Combine supplements for optimal health benefits.

Supplement stacking, a strategy widely employed in the biohacking community, involves combining various dietary supplements to achieve optimal health benefits. This approach is based on the idea that certain supplements can work synergistically, enhancing each other's effects. Dr. Rhonda Patrick, a biomedical scientist known for her research on nutritional health, notes, "Strategically combining supplements can enhance their individual benefits, leading to improved overall health outcomes" (Patrick, 2018). Patrick's research and advocacy have helped popularize the concept of supplement stacking for enhanced health benefits.

A common example of supplement stacking is the combination of magnesium, zinc, and vitamin B6, known as ZMA, often used to improve sleep quality and muscle recovery. Another popular stack combines omega-3 fatty acids, vitamin D, and curcumin for improved joint health and inflammation reduction. "The right combination of supplements can target specific health goals more effectively than single supplements alone," says Dr. Michael Murray, a naturopathic doctor and expert in natural medicine (Murray, 2017).

While supplement stacking can offer enhanced health benefits, it requires careful consideration of the individual supplements' compatibility and dosages. It's important for individuals to research and potentially consult with health professionals to ensure safe and effective use. Supplement stacking exemplifies a proactive and personalized approach to health and wellness, characteristic of the biohacking ethos.

Cryotherapy: Use extreme cold for recovery and inflammation reduction.

Cryotherapy, a popular biohacking method, involves the use of extreme cold temperatures for short periods to aid in recovery and reduce inflammation. This technique, often used by athletes and fitness enthusiasts, exposes the body to subzero temperatures, triggering physiological responses that can lead to various health benefits. Dr. Rhonda Patrick, known for her research in health and longevity, states, "Cryotherapy can significantly reduce inflammation and improve recovery time by stimulating cold receptors in the skin, which send signals to the brain to initiate anti-inflammatory responses" (Patrick, 2016). Her research underscores the effectiveness of cryotherapy in managing inflammation and speeding up recovery.

The process typically involves standing in a cryotherapy chamber for two to four minutes, where temperatures can drop as low as -140 degrees Celsius (-220 degrees Fahrenheit). This exposure to extreme cold causes blood vessels to constrict, reducing blood flow to areas of inflammation and pain. Upon exiting the chamber, blood vessels expand, and blood flow increases, flushing away toxins and supplying nutrients and oxygen to the body. "Cryotherapy can be a powerful tool to alleviate muscle soreness and improve overall well-being," explains Dr. Joseph Mercola, an advocate for alternative health practices (Mercola, 2017).

Cryotherapy has been adopted not only for physical recovery but also for its potential benefits in mood enhancement, skin rejuvenation, and weight loss. However, it's important for individuals to approach cryotherapy with caution, especially those with certain health conditions. This biohacking practice represents an advanced approach to health and wellness, leveraging the body's natural responses to extreme temperatures for therapeutic benefits.

Biofeedback Training: Learn to control body functions like heart rate.

Biofeedback training, a technique embraced by the biohacking community, involves using technology to gain control over bodily functions typically considered involuntary, like heart rate, muscle tension, and skin temperature. This method provides real-time feedback about physiological functions, allowing individuals to learn how to make subtle changes to their body, such as relaxing certain muscles or reducing stress. Dr. Erik Peper, a renowned biofeedback researcher, states, "Biofeedback training enables an individual to learn how to change physiological activity for the purposes of improving health and performance" (Peper, 2014). This approach underscores the power of awareness and self-regulation in enhancing personal well-being.

Biofeedback devices measure various physiological parameters and relay this information back to the user, often through a computer or mobile app. This feedback helps users recognize and modify their physiological responses to stress, anxiety, or physical discomfort. "Biofeedback can be particularly effective in treating conditions exacerbated by stress, such as migraine headaches, high blood pressure, and chronic pain," explains Dr. Richard Gevirtz, a leader in biofeedback research (Gevirtz, 2015).

Adopting biofeedback training as part of a health and wellness regimen allows individuals to take an active role in managing their health. This practice aligns with the biohacking principle of using data and technology to improve one's physical and mental performance. Biofeedback training exemplifies a proactive approach to health, providing tools and techniques to enhance self-awareness and control over one's own bodily functions.

Virtual Reality Meditation: Use VR for immersive relaxation experiences.

Virtual Reality (VR) Meditation, a novel biohacking trend, combines the immersive technology of VR with the ancient practice of meditation to create unique relaxation experiences. By using VR headsets, users are transported into serene, digitally-created environments, which can range from tranquil beaches to mystical forests. This innovative approach to meditation can significantly enhance the depth and quality of the experience. Dr. Brennan Spiegel, Director of Health Services Research at Cedars-Sinai, explains, "VR can be more effective than traditional meditation practices for some people because it immersively distracts them from their immediate surroundings, helping to reduce anxiety and stress" (Spiegel, 2018). His research highlights the potential of VR as a powerful tool in mental health and relaxation.

The immersive nature of VR meditation allows users to shut out external distractions more effectively, facilitating a deeper state of mindfulness and relaxation. By engaging multiple senses, VR meditation can create a more focused and guided experience, beneficial for beginners who might struggle with traditional meditation practices. "Virtual reality can guide users through meditation exercises in a highly controlled and effective way," states Dr. Giuseppe

Riva, a researcher in cyberpsychology and eHealth (Riva, 2017).

VR meditation represents an intersection of technology and wellness, offering a modern twist to traditional relaxation techniques. This biohack caters to the increasing need for effective stress-management tools in our fast-paced world, providing a unique and accessible approach to achieving calmness and mental clarity.

Plant-Based Diet: Explore health benefits of vegetarianism or veganism.

A plant-based diet, emphasizing the consumption of vegetables, fruits, grains, nuts, and seeds while excluding or minimizing animal products, has gained significant traction in the biohacking community for its health benefits. This dietary approach, encompassing vegetarianism and veganism, is lauded for its potential in reducing the risk of chronic diseases, improving heart health, and aiding weight management. Dr. Dean Ornish, a clinical professor of medicine and an advocate for plant-based diets, states, "A plant-based diet can not only prevent but also reverse some of the top killer diseases in the modern world, including heart disease, type 2 diabetes, and high blood pressure" (Ornish, 2019). His extensive research provides compelling evidence for the health advantages of a diet rich in plant-based foods.

The core principle of a plant-based diet is to derive most of the nutritional needs from plant sources. This approach is not just about eliminating meat; it's about focusing on whole, minimally processed plants that are rich in vitamins, minerals, fiber, and antioxidants. Dr. T. Colin Campbell, a biochemist and author renowned for his work on the dietary connection to chronic diseases, emphasizes, "The whole foods, plant-based diet provides the most health-promoting and disease-fighting nutrients. It consists of foods that are natural and minimally processed" (Campbell, 2005).

Adopting a plant-based diet as a biohack goes beyond individual health. It also addresses environmental concerns and ethical considerations about animal welfare. However, it requires careful planning to ensure all nutritional needs, particularly protein, iron, calcium, and B vitamins, are met. As a dietary approach, vegetarianism and veganism offer a pathway not only towards improved personal health but also towards a more sustainable and ethical way of living.

DIY Fermentation: Make probiotic-rich foods like kombucha or sauerkraut.

DIY Fermentation, a practice embraced by the biohacking community, involves the homemade creation of probiotic-rich foods like kombucha, sauerkraut, and yogurt. This process harnesses the power of natural fermentation to cultivate beneficial bacteria, enhancing gut health and overall well-being. Sandor Katz, a fermentation revivalist and author, advocates for the practice: "Fermentation not only preserves nutrients but also breaks them down into more easily digestible forms. The live cultures created during fermentation can replenish the microbiome, contributing to a healthy gut" (Katz, 2012). Katz's work has been instrumental in popularizing fermentation as a healthful and accessible practice.

Fermenting at home is a simple and cost-effective way to produce foods rich in probiotics, enzymes, and vitamins.

Kombucha, a fermented tea, has gained popularity for its tangy flavor and health benefits, including improved digestion and immune support. Sauerkraut, fermented cabbage, is known for its high vitamin C and probiotic content. "The beauty of fermentation is its simplicity and the connection it gives us to the microbial world," notes Dr. Joseph Mercola, an advocate for natural health practices (Mercola, 2013).

DIY fermentation is more than just a means to produce nutritious foods; it's a return to traditional food preparation methods, offering control over what goes into the food we consume. This biohack not only benefits physical health but also fosters a deeper understanding and appreciation of the role of bacteria in our diets and lives.

UV Exposure Tracking: Monitor and optimize Vitamin D synthesis.

UV Exposure Tracking, a biohacking practice gaining momentum, involves monitoring one's exposure to ultraviolet (UV) light to optimize Vitamin D synthesis, essential for bone health, immune function, and overall well-being. This approach is particularly significant in a world where lifestyles often limit time spent outdoors, leading to potential Vitamin D deficiencies. Dr. Michael Holick, a professor of medicine and a leading expert on Vitamin D research, emphasizes the importance of UV exposure for Vitamin D production: "Sensible sun exposure, especially between 10 AM and 3 PM, with about 40% of your skin exposed, can provide a healthy dose of Vitamin D" (Holick, 2017). Holick's guidelines highlight the balance needed between obtaining Vitamin D and minimizing the risk of skin damage.

Modern UV exposure tracking devices, ranging from wearable tech to smartphone apps, help individuals gauge their exposure to UV light. These tools provide insights into the optimal duration and intensity of sunlight needed to maintain adequate Vitamin D levels without overexposure. "Understanding your UV exposure is crucial for maintaining skin health while also reaping the benefits of Vitamin D," notes Dr. Nina Jablonski, an anthropologist specializing in skin and sunlight (Jablonski, 2018).

Incorporating UV exposure tracking into daily life represents a proactive approach to health. It not only helps optimize Vitamin D synthesis but also raises awareness about skin cancer risks associated with excessive sun exposure. This biohacking method exemplifies a data-driven approach to health, enabling individuals to make informed decisions about their sun exposure for optimal health benefits.

Sensory Deprivation Tanks: Experience flotation therapy for relaxation.

Sensory Deprivation Tanks, also known as flotation therapy, offer a unique experience in the biohacking world for achieving deep relaxation and mental clarity. These tanks, filled with saltwater, are designed to minimize sensory input to the brain, including light, sound, and tactile sensations. The high salt concentration allows individuals to float effortlessly, creating a feeling of weightlessness. Dr. Peter Suedfeld, a pioneer in REST (Restricted Environmental Stimulation Therapy) research, explains, "Flotation therapy can induce a deep state of relaxation and a tranquil mind, helping reduce stress and anxiety levels" (Suedfeld, 1980). His research indicates significant psychological and physiological benefits from sensory deprivation experiences.

The buoyancy achieved in these tanks reduces the strain on the body, particularly on the spine and joints, facilitating physical relaxation and pain relief. The minimal sensory input allows the mind to drift into a meditative state, promoting mental recovery and creativity. Joe Rogan, a prominent advocate of flotation therapy, describes the experience: "It's the most bizarre and cool feeling to just float in space and not feel your body" (Rogan, 2014). Rogan's endorsement reflects the growing popularity of flotation therapy for mental and physical wellness.

Flotation therapy in sensory deprivation tanks is more than a relaxation technique; it's a form of biohacking that leverages the absence of stimuli to promote mental and physical well-being. This practice provides a unique environment for individuals to disconnect from external sensory overload and explore the depths of their own consciousness, offering profound relaxation and self-discovery benefits.

Electronic Muscle Stimulation (EMS): Enhance muscle activation and recovery.

Electronic Muscle Stimulation (EMS), a method increasingly utilized in the biohacking community, employs electrical impulses to enhance muscle activation and recovery. This technique is particularly beneficial for athletes and fitness enthusiasts seeking to improve muscle strength, endurance, and repair. Dr. John Porcari, a professor of exercise and sports science, highlights EMS's efficacy, stating, "EMS can be used as a training, therapeutic, or cosmetic tool, enhancing muscle strength and recovery after workouts" (Porcari, 2011). Porcari's research demonstrates EMS's versatility in fitness and rehabilitation settings.

EMS works by sending low-level electrical currents through electrodes placed on the skin, directly above the muscles to be stimulated. These currents mimic the action potential coming from the central nervous system, causing the muscles to contract. This method can target specific muscle groups, enhancing the effectiveness of strength training and rehabilitation exercises. "EMS can activate muscles more effectively than voluntary contractions alone," asserts Dr. Nicola Maffiuletti, a specialist in neuromuscular research (Maffiuletti, 2016).

The use of EMS is not only limited to enhancing workout efficiency; it also plays a crucial role in injury prevention and recovery. By stimulating muscles that may not be effectively activated through conventional exercise, EMS helps in balancing muscle strength and reducing the risk of injury. This biohacking tool exemplifies the integration of technology in health and fitness, offering an advanced approach to muscle development and recovery.

Breathwork Techniques: Practice methods like Wim Hof for energy and health.

Breathwork Techniques, particularly methods like the Wim Hof Method, have gained significant attention in the biohacking community for their ability to enhance energy, health, and resilience. This practice involves controlled breathing exercises that significantly impact the autonomic nervous system and immune response. Wim Hof, known as "The Iceman" for his ability to withstand extreme cold, describes the essence of his method: "Proper breathing can change your life, and increase your energy, health, and well-being" (Hof, 2020). Hof's method combines specific breathing techniques with cold exposure and meditation to improve physical and mental health.

The Wim Hof Method's breathing exercises involve a cycle of controlled hyperventilation followed by breath retention. This process is believed to alkalize the body, reduce stress, and enhance concentration and mental clarity. Research led by Dr. Matthijs Kox, a physiologist, found that individuals trained in the Wim Hof Method could influence their autonomic nervous system and immune response, previously thought to be beyond voluntary control (Kox, 2014). This groundbreaking discovery underscores the potential of breathwork in managing physiological responses.

Adopting breathwork techniques as a biohack offers a powerful tool for enhancing overall well-being. These practices do not require special equipment and can be incorporated into daily routines, making them accessible to a wide audience. Breathwork stands out for its ability to improve physical performance, mental clarity, and emotional resilience, aligning with the biohacking ethos of self-optimization and holistic health.

Microdosing: Explore microdosing of certain substances for cognitive benefits.

Microdosing, a practice gaining traction in the biohacking community, involves taking minimal amounts of certain substances, often psychedelics like LSD or psilocybin, to achieve cognitive and emotional benefits without experiencing a full-blown psychedelic trip. This approach is said to enhance creativity, productivity, and emotional insight while maintaining normal functioning. Dr. James Fadiman, a psychologist known for his work on psychedelic research, explains, "Microdosing provides the possibility for cognitive and emotional improvement without the intensity of a full psychedelic experience" (Fadiman, 2011). Fadiman's research suggests potential benefits in mood enhancement and problem-solving abilities.

The principle behind microdosing is that sub-perceptual doses, typically around one-tenth of a recreational dose, can subtly influence thought patterns and mood without significant alterations in perception. Users report improved mood, heightened awareness, and increased creativity. "Microdosing can offer a new form of therapy, providing benefits like enhanced mood and increased focus," states Dr. Robin Carhart-Harris, head of the Centre for Psychedelic Research at Imperial College London (Carhart-Harris, 2019).

While microdosing shows promise, it remains a legally and scientifically grey area, with more research needed to fully understand its effects and implications. It represents a cutting-edge biohacking practice, pushing the boundaries of conventional approaches to cognitive enhancement and emotional well-being. As with any substance use, caution and informed decision-making are paramount.

Grounding or Earthing: Connect with nature to reduce inflammation.

Grounding or Earthing, a practice increasingly embraced by the biohacking community, involves direct contact with the Earth's surface, such as walking barefoot on grass or sand, to harness natural healing energy. This connection is believed to reduce inflammation, improve sleep, and enhance overall well-being. Dr. James Oschman, a biophysicist and pioneer in the field of Earthing, states, "Connecting to the Earth's electrical energy can have healing effects, including reduced pain and inflammation" (Oschman, 2009). His research highlights the physiological changes that occur with direct contact with the Earth.

The theory behind grounding is that the Earth possesses a negative electrical potential and that by making direct contact, the body can absorb negative electrons. These electrons are thought to neutralize free radicals, which are positively charged and known to contribute to inflammation and disease. "Grounding can be a simple, yet profoundly effective strategy for reducing inflammation and pain in the body," explains Dr. Stephen Sinatra, a cardiologist and proponent of Earthing (Sinatra, 2011).

Incorporating grounding into daily life represents a return to a more natural and harmonious way of living. This practice encourages individuals to reconnect with nature, offering a simple and accessible means to potentially reduce chronic inflammation and promote health and vitality. Grounding exemplifies a biohacking approach that is both ancestral and innovative, utilizing the Earth's innate properties for health enhancement.

Acupressure Mats: Use for pain relief and relaxation.

Acupressure Mats, an increasingly popular tool in the biohacking community, offer a simple yet effective method for pain relief and relaxation. These mats are covered with thousands of small, sharp spikes that stimulate acupressure points across the back and body. The principle behind their use is akin to acupuncture but without needles. Dr. Michael Reed Gach, an acupressure specialist, explains, "Acupressure mats work by stimulating specific points on the body, which releases endorphins and blocks pain signals to the brain" (Gach, 2010). Gach's insight points to the effectiveness of acupressure in managing pain and promoting relaxation.

Lying on an acupressure mat for just 20-30 minutes a day can trigger the body's natural healing responses. The spikes on the mat increase blood flow and oxygen to the area, which can help reduce muscle tension and pain. Many users report improvements in headaches, back pain, insomnia, and stress levels. "Regular use of acupressure mats can lead to better sleep, reduced stress, and improved energy levels," states Dr. Karen Sherman, a researcher in alternative medicine (Sherman, 2013).

Acupressure mats embody a convenient and non-invasive approach to pain management and relaxation, aligning with the biohacking ethos of using simple, natural methods to enhance health. Their growing popularity is a testament to their effectiveness in providing relief and promoting well-being.

Smart Water Bottles: Track hydration levels.

Smart Water Bottles, a modern innovation embraced by the biohacking community, are designed to track hydration levels, reminding users to drink water regularly to maintain optimal hydration. Equipped with sensors and connected to apps, these bottles monitor water intake and provide data-driven insights into one's hydration habits. Dr. Alexis C. Wood, a nutrition scientist, emphasizes the importance of hydration, stating, "Proper hydration is crucial for maintaining bodily functions, including brain function, heart rate, and metabolism" (Wood, 2019). Her research highlights the critical role of water in overall health.

These bottles often feature reminders, either in the form of lights or through smartphone notifications, prompting users to drink water at regular intervals. This technology is particularly beneficial for those who lead busy lives and may forget to stay adequately hydrated. "Smart water bottles can be a practical solution for people to track their water intake and ensure they are staying hydrated throughout the day," explains Dr. Dana Cohen, an expert in integrative medicine (Cohen, 2018).

Incorporating a smart water bottle into one's daily routine represents a simple yet effective biohack for maintaining hydration, a fundamental aspect of health often overlooked. This tool exemplifies how technology can be leveraged to support health and wellness, offering a user-friendly and interactive approach to staying hydrated.

Personalized Vitamin Regimens: Tailor supplements to individual needs.

Personalized Vitamin Regimens, a concept widely adopted in the biohacking community, involve customizing supplement intake based on individual health needs, lifestyle, and sometimes genetic profiles. This tailored approach ensures that individuals receive the specific nutrients they require for optimal health, as opposed to the one-size-fits-all solution offered by standard multivitamins. Dr. Pieter Cohen, an associate professor of medicine, emphasizes the importance of personalized nutrition, stating, "Customizing vitamin and supplement regimens to individual needs can significantly improve health outcomes by addressing specific deficiencies and health goals" (Cohen, 2015). Cohen's insight highlights the shift towards more individualized health care and wellness strategies.

Personalized regimens often begin with a detailed assessment, which may include blood tests, genetic testing, and lifestyle evaluations, to identify specific nutritional gaps and needs. This approach is particularly beneficial for addressing unique health concerns, supporting athletic performance, or managing chronic conditions. "Tailored vitamin regimens can be more effective than generic supplements, as they are based on the individual's unique health profile," explains Dr. Michael Roizen, a wellness expert (Roizen, 2016).

Adopting a personalized vitamin regimen represents a proactive and data-driven approach to health and wellness. It aligns with the biohacking principle of optimizing one's body based on personal health data and scientific research, ensuring that supplementation is both effective and appropriate for the individual's specific health requirements.

Aromatherapy: Use essential oils for mood and health benefits.

Aromatherapy, a practice embraced by the biohacking community, utilizes essential oils extracted from plants for their therapeutic properties to enhance mood and health. This holistic treatment leverages the powerful scents of essential oils to stimulate the limbic system, the part of the brain that plays a key role in emotions, behaviors, and long-term memory. Dr. Axe, a natural medicine advocate, explains, "Aromatherapy works by stimulating smell receptors in the nose, which then send messages through the nervous system to the limbic system — the part of the brain that controls emotions" (Axe, 2017). This connection highlights the potential of aromatherapy in influencing psychological well-being.

Essential oils like lavender, peppermint, and eucalyptus are popular in aromatherapy for their varied benefits. Lavender is renowned for its calming and relaxing effects, often used to alleviate stress and improve sleep. Peppermint oil is praised for its invigorating and pain-relief properties, while eucalyptus oil is known for its respiratory benefits. "Lavender oil has been shown to reduce anxiety and improve sleep quality in patients with anxiety disorders and sleep disturbances," states Dr. Janmejai K Srivastava, a researcher in complementary medicine (Srivastava, 2010).

Incorporating aromatherapy into daily routines can be done through diffusers, aromatic spritzers, inhalers, bathing salts, body oils, creams, or clay masks. This practice offers a natural and non-invasive way to enhance emotional and physical well-being, exemplifying the biohacking ethos of leveraging natural resources for health optimization.

Infrared Saunas: Detoxify and relax with deep heat.

Infrared Saunas, increasingly popular in the biohacking community, utilize infrared heaters to emit radiant heat absorbed directly by the body, offering a deep, detoxifying sweat at lower temperatures than traditional saunas. This form of sauna therapy is celebrated for its ability to relax muscles, relieve pain, and purge toxins from the body. Dr.

Lawrence Wilson, an advocate for sauna therapy, states, "Infrared saunas help the body sweat out toxins and heavy metals, and they can be more effective than traditional saunas due to the deeper penetration of infrared light" (Wilson, 2014). His research suggests a significant detoxification effect that surpasses conventional sauna methods.

The deep penetration of infrared heat stimulates the cardiovascular, lymphatic, and immune systems, increasing blood flow and promoting a more intense detoxifying sweat. This process not only helps in eliminating toxins but also aids in muscle relaxation and stress reduction. "Regular use of infrared saunas can lead to improved circulation, relaxation, and general well-being," notes Dr. Richard Beever, a clinical assistant professor who has researched the health benefits of saunas (Beever, 2009).

Incorporating infrared sauna sessions into a wellness routine is a biohacking strategy that aligns with the pursuit of holistic health. It offers a comforting, relaxing experience while providing substantial health benefits, including detoxification, pain relief, and improved circulation, making it a valuable tool in the biohacker's toolkit for health optimization.

Sound Therapy: Use binaural beats for relaxation and focus.

Sound Therapy, particularly through the use of binaural beats, is a biohacking technique that involves listening to sound frequencies to induce states of relaxation, focus, or even sleep. Binaural beats occur when slightly different frequencies are played in each ear, creating a third tone that the brain perceives, which can influence brainwave patterns. Dr. Gerald Oster, a biophysicist who contributed to the early understanding of binaural beats, explains, "Binaural beats can be used to induce certain mental states, as different frequencies can influence brain wave patterns" (Oster, 1973). His research opened the door to the therapeutic use of binaural beats in managing stress, anxiety, and cognitive function.

When listening to binaural beats, the brain aligns with the frequency difference, known as the 'beat,' potentially leading to enhanced focus, relaxation, or meditation states, depending on the frequency used. "Binaural beats in the delta and theta range have been shown to induce a relaxation response and can improve sleep quality," says Dr. Bruce Tainio, a specialist in frequency therapy (Tainio, 1999).

Using binaural beats as a biohacking tool involves listening to these auditory illusions with headphones to ensure each ear receives a slightly different frequency. This practice is increasingly popular for its simplicity and non-invasive approach to improving mental states. Whether for deepening meditation, enhancing concentration, or promoting better sleep, sound therapy with binaural beats offers a unique and accessible means of achieving specific mental states.

Oxygen Therapy/Training: Enhance performance and recovery.

Oxygen Therapy/Training, a technique increasingly utilized in the biohacking community, involves breathing in pure or enriched oxygen to enhance physical performance, accelerate recovery, and improve overall wellness. This method is based on the principle that increasing oxygen intake can significantly improve the efficiency of oxygen utilization in the body. Dr. Richard Levitan, an emergency physician and advocate for oxygen therapy, notes, "Oxygen therapy can significantly boost athletic performance and aid in faster recovery by enhancing tissue oxygenation" (Levitan, 2020). Levitan's insights reflect the growing interest in oxygen therapy as a tool for health optimization.

This practice is commonly used by athletes to increase endurance, speed up recovery, and enhance performance. It's also beneficial in medical settings for treating conditions like chronic obstructive pulmonary disease (COPD) and promoting faster healing of wounds. "Hyperbaric oxygen therapy, which involves breathing pure oxygen in a pressurized room or chamber, is known for accelerating wound healing and improving the body's natural healing processes," explains Dr. Paul Harch, a pioneer in hyperbaric medicine (Harch, 2017).

Adopting oxygen therapy/training as part of a health and fitness regimen represents a biohacking strategy aimed at maximizing the body's potential. Whether through high-oxygen-content environments or supplemental oxygen during workouts, this approach exemplifies the biohacking ethos of enhancing physical capabilities and recovery through innovative and scientifically-backed methods.

Herbal Nootropics: Experiment with natural cognitive enhancers.

Herbal Nootropics, a key interest in the biohacking community, involve the use of natural supplements derived from plants to enhance cognitive functions such as memory, creativity, and focus. These botanicals offer a holistic approach to boosting brain power, often with fewer side effects than synthetic nootropics. Dr. Ray Sahelian, a physician and author specializing in natural supplements, states, "Herbal nootropics, like ginkgo biloba and bacopa monnieri, have been shown to enhance brain function and mental clarity" (Sahelian, 2015). His research underscores the potential of these natural substances in cognitive enhancement.

Ginkgo biloba, for instance, is renowned for its ability to improve blood flow to the brain and enhance cognitive function, while bacopa monnieri is praised for its memory-enhancing and neuroprotective properties. Ashwagandha, another popular herbal nootropic, is known for reducing stress and anxiety, in addition to improving brain function. "Adaptogenic herbs like ashwagandha can not only help improve focus and mental stamina but also regulate the body's response to stress," explains Dr. Brenda Powell, a specialist in integrative medicine (Powell, 2016).

Incorporating herbal nootropics into a daily wellness routine represents a biohacking approach that aligns with a preference for natural, holistic health strategies. These botanicals offer a way to enhance cognitive function and manage stress, while potentially supporting overall brain health. As with any supplement, it's important for individuals to research and consult healthcare professionals to ensure safety and efficacy.

Biohacking Spaces/Environments: Design living spaces for optimal health.

Biohacking Spaces/Environments, an emerging trend in the biohacking community, involves designing living and working spaces that promote optimal health and well-being. This approach recognizes that our surroundings significantly impact our physical and mental health. Dr. Esther Sternberg, a researcher in environmental health, notes, "The spaces we inhabit can influence our mood, immune function, and overall health" (Sternberg, 2009). Her work highlights the profound effect of our physical environment on our well-being.

This concept extends to various aspects of space design, including lighting, air quality, ergonomics, and even the presence of natural elements like plants. For example, using full-spectrum light bulbs can mimic natural sunlight, helping regulate circadian rhythms and improve mood. "Good lighting design can boost your energy during the day and improve your sleep at night," explains Dr. Mark Rea, a professor specializing in light and health (Rea, 2012).

Creating biohacking spaces is about more than aesthetics; it's about constructing environments that actively contribute to health and productivity. This might involve air purifying systems to improve air quality, ergonomic furniture to prevent posture-related issues, or the strategic use of color to influence mood and energy levels. By incorporating these elements, biohacking spaces aim to create environments that support and enhance the body's natural functioning and well-being.

Virtual Fitness Coaching: Personalized training via AI or online platforms.

Virtual Fitness Coaching, a rapidly growing trend in the biohacking community, leverages artificial intelligence (AI) and online platforms to offer personalized training programs. This technology-driven approach allows individuals to access tailored workout plans, nutritional advice, and progress tracking tools from the comfort of their homes. Dr. John P. Higgins, a sports cardiologist, explains, "Virtual fitness coaching can provide customized training and feedback that adapts to an individual's progress and goals" (Higgins, 2018). Higgins' insights reflect the increasing demand for personalized and accessible fitness solutions.

AI-driven fitness platforms use algorithms to analyze a user's fitness level, preferences, and goals to create a customized workout regimen. These platforms can adjust training plans based on the user's progress, providing a dynamic and responsive fitness experience. "The advantage of AI in fitness coaching is its ability to learn from your performance and continuously adapt the training to optimize results," notes Dr. Jennifer B. Ullrich, a researcher in health technologies (Ullrich, 2019).

Virtual fitness coaching offers the flexibility of working out anytime and anywhere, making it an attractive option for those with busy schedules or limited access to traditional gym facilities. It represents a fusion of technology and fitness, aligning with the biohacking principle of using data-driven approaches to enhance physical health and performance. This modern approach to fitness coaching exemplifies the evolving landscape of health and wellness in the digital age.

Adaptogen Supplements: Manage stress and fatigue with natural herbs.

Adaptogen Supplements, increasingly popular in the biohacking community, involve the use of natural herbs that help the body manage stress and combat fatigue. Adaptogens, a unique class of herbal ingredients, are known for their ability to balance, restore, and protect the body. Dr. Brenda Powell, co-medical director of the Center for Integrative and Lifestyle Medicine, elaborates, "Adaptogens help your body handle stress. They work at a molecular level by regulating a stable balance in the hypothalamic, pituitary, and adrenal glands" (Powell, 2018). Her statement underscores the holistic impact of adaptogens on the body's stress response systems.

Common adaptogens include herbs like ashwagandha, Rhodiola rosea, and ginseng. Ashwagandha is renowned for its ability to reduce cortisol levels and combat the effects of stress. Rhodiola rosea is often used for enhancing mental performance and alleviating fatigue. Ginseng is praised for its energy-boosting and immune-enhancing properties. "Adaptogens like Rhodiola rosea can significantly reduce fatigue and improve cognitive function during periods of stress," explains Dr. Patricia Gerbarg, an assistant clinical professor in psychiatry (Gerbarg, 2017).

Incorporating adaptogen supplements into a daily wellness routine can provide a natural, effective way to manage stress and improve energy levels. This approach aligns with the biohacking ethos of leveraging natural substances to enhance the body's resilience and optimize health. As with any supplement, it's important for individuals to consult with healthcare professionals to ensure safety and suitability for their specific health needs.

Custom Orthotics: Improve posture and walking patterns.

Custom Orthotics, a solution increasingly adopted by the biohacking community, involves the use of specially designed shoe inserts to improve posture, walking patterns, and overall musculoskeletal health. These orthotics are tailored to the specific contours and biomechanics of an individual's feet, providing support where it's needed most. Dr. Kevin Kirby, a podiatrist and adjunct associate professor, states, "Custom orthotics are designed to correct your specific foot imbalances, reduce stress and strain on your body, and bring your feet back into proper alignment" (Kirby, 2016). Kirby's insights emphasize the importance of addressing foot biomechanics for overall physical health.

Custom orthotics work by aligning the foot and ankle into the most anatomically efficient position, thereby alleviating stress on the joints and muscles of the foot, leg, and lower back. This can lead to a reduction in pain and improvement in function. "Orthotics can play a crucial role in preventing injuries and enhancing comfort for people who spend long hours on their feet or have specific foot conditions," explains Dr. Howard Dananberg, a specialist in gait and foot function (Dananberg, 2014).

Using custom orthotics is more than just a remedy for foot-related issues; it's a proactive approach to enhancing overall body mechanics and well-being. These devices exemplify the biohacking principle of personalizing health solutions to meet individual needs, offering a tailored approach to improving posture and physical performance.

Quantified Self Movement: Track personal data for life optimization.

The Quantified Self Movement, embraced by the biohacking community, centers around the tracking of personal data to optimize various aspects of life, including health, fitness, productivity, and sleep. This self-tracking is achieved through a range of technologies like wearables, smartphone apps, and specialized sensors. Gary Wolf, a journalist and co-founder of the Quantified Self Movement, describes its essence: "It's about self-knowledge through self-tracking with technology" (Wolf, 2010). Wolf's definition underscores the movement's focus on data-driven approaches to personal improvement.

Participants in the Quantified Self Movement meticulously collect and analyze data about their daily activities and bodily functions to identify patterns, trends, and areas for improvement. From monitoring heart rate variability and sleep patterns to tracking exercise, nutrition, and mental health, the movement empowers individuals to take a data-driven approach to enhance their well-being. "By quantifying personal data, we can make better decisions about our health, habits, and routines," explains Dr. Deborah Lupton, a sociologist specializing in the quantified self and health (Lupton, 2016).

The Quantified Self Movement represents a shift towards more personalized and informed approaches to health and lifestyle optimization. It aligns with the biohacking ethos of experimentation, self-discovery, and using technology to improve one's quality of life. This movement exemplifies a proactive and empowered approach to personal health and well-being in the digital age.

Peptides for Healing and Performance: Explore peptide therapy.

Peptides for Healing and Performance, a rapidly growing interest within the biohacking community, involve the use of specific amino acid sequences, known as peptides, for therapeutic purposes. These peptides are used to promote healing, enhance physical performance, and improve overall health. Dr. Daniel Stickler, a physician and expert in peptide therapy, explains, "Peptides can play a crucial role in a wide range of bodily functions, from muscle growth and fat loss to anti-aging and tissue repair" (Stickler, 2018). His insights highlight the versatile and powerful nature of peptide therapy in health optimization.

Peptides, naturally occurring in the body, can be synthesized and administered to target specific areas of health. For instance, BPC-157, a peptide known for its healing properties, is used to accelerate wound healing and reduce inflammation. Another peptide, CJC-1295, is popular for its growth hormone-releasing properties, enhancing muscle growth and overall vitality. "The targeted use of peptides can support the body's natural healing processes and optimize physical performance," states Dr. William Seeds, a leading researcher in peptide therapy (Seeds, 2019).

Incorporating peptide therapy into health and wellness routines is becoming an increasingly popular biohack for those seeking advanced methods to enhance healing and physical capabilities. This approach represents a cutting-edge frontier in biohacking, where science and health converge to offer tailored solutions for longevity, recovery, and performance enhancement.

Smart Sleep Alarms: Wake up at the optimal sleep phase.

Smart Sleep Alarms, a technology embraced by the biohacking community, are designed to wake individuals during the optimal phase of their sleep cycle, aiming to reduce grogginess and improve overall sleep quality. These alarms work by monitoring sleep patterns, either through wearable devices or smartphone apps, and identifying the lightest sleep phase within a designated wake-up window. Dr. Rebecca Robbins, a sleep researcher at Harvard Medical School, states, "Waking up during a lighter sleep phase can help you feel more refreshed and alert upon awakening" (Robbins, 2018). Robbins' research supports the idea that the timing of waking up is crucial for how rested an individual feels.

Unlike traditional alarms that may abruptly awaken an individual during deep sleep, smart sleep alarms aim to wake the user during lighter sleep stages, such as REM or light sleep. This method can significantly enhance the waking experience, making it feel more natural and less jarring. "Smart sleep alarms can be a useful tool for those seeking to optimize their sleep and wake up feeling more rested," explains Dr. Matthew Walker, a professor of neuroscience and psychology and author of "Why We Sleep" (Walker, 2017).

Incorporating smart sleep alarms into a sleep routine represents a biohacking strategy focused on enhancing sleep quality and overall well-being. This approach exemplifies the use of technology to align with the body's natural rhythms, offering a sophisticated solution to improve sleep and, consequently, daily performance and health.

Neurofeedback for ADHD: Manage attention disorders through brain training.

Neurofeedback for ADHD, a method increasingly utilized in the biohacking and therapeutic communities, involves brain training exercises to help manage Attention Deficit Hyperactivity Disorder (ADHD). This non-invasive technique uses real-time displays of brain activity, often through EEG, to teach individuals how to regulate their own brain function. Dr. Joel Lubar, a pioneer in the use of neurofeedback for ADHD, explains, "Neurofeedback trains individuals to alter their brain waves, which can lead to improvements in focus, impulsivity, and hyperactivity in ADHD" (Lubar, 1995). Lubar's research has been instrumental in validating neurofeedback as an effective tool for managing ADHD symptoms.

During neurofeedback sessions, individuals with ADHD learn to recognize and modify their brainwave patterns associated with focus and concentration. This process can lead to a reduction in ADHD symptoms and an improvement in attention span, impulse control, and overall mental clarity. "Neurofeedback offers a promising alternative for individuals seeking non-pharmacological treatment options for ADHD," states Dr. Hallowell, a psychiatrist and ADHD expert (Hallowell, 2010).

Adopting neurofeedback as a biohacking practice for ADHD management represents a shift towards more personalized and empowering approaches to mental health. It aligns with the biohacking ethos of using data-driven techniques to enhance cognitive functioning and well-being. Neurofeedback for ADHD exemplifies a practical application of neuroscience in improving everyday life for those with attention disorders.

Genetic Editing (CRISPR): Explore the future potential of genetic modification.

Genetic Editing, particularly through the use of CRISPR (Clustered Regularly Interspaced Short Palindromic Repeats) technology, represents a frontier in biohacking, offering the potential for precise genetic modification. CRISPR allows scientists to edit genomes with unprecedented precision, efficiency, and flexibility. Dr. Jennifer Doudna, a biochemist and co-developer of CRISPR-Cas9 technology, states, "CRISPR technology is a tool that can be used to edit genes. In the future, it could be used to treat genetic disorders and diseases" (Doudna, 2015). Doudna's groundbreaking work has opened up new possibilities in genetic research and therapeutics.

CRISPR technology works by using an enzyme, typically Cas9, guided by a piece of RNA designed to match the sequence of a specific gene. This system can cut the DNA at the targeted location, allowing for the removal, addition, or alteration of specific genetic sequences. "CRISPR could revolutionize how we treat and prevent many diseases, offering possibilities that were unimaginable a few years ago," explains Dr. Feng Zhang, a molecular biologist instrumental in the development of CRISPR technology (Zhang, 2014).

The potential applications of CRISPR are vast, from correcting genetic defects to improving crop resilience. However, the ethical and safety implications of gene editing are subjects of intense debate. As the technology continues to develop, it represents a significant area of interest in biohacking and scientific communities, embodying the cutting-edge of efforts to understand and manipulate the fundamental codes of life for health and disease management.

Mind-Machine Interfaces: Experiment with technology to enhance cognitive abilities.

Mind-Machine Interfaces (MMIs), a rapidly advancing area in the biohacking community, involve the use of technology to directly connect the human brain with external devices to enhance cognitive abilities. These interfaces, which can include brain-computer interfaces (BCIs) and neuroprosthetics, allow for direct communication between the brain and a machine, bypassing the need for traditional motor pathways. Dr. Miguel Nicolelis, a neuroscientist known for his work on MMIs, explains, "Mind-machine interfaces can decode neural signals and translate them into actions, enabling new ways to interact with technology" (Nicolelis, 2011). His pioneering research has contributed to the development of technologies that can augment human capabilities.

MMIs have the potential to revolutionize how we interact with computers, control prosthetic limbs, and even restore functions lost due to neurological disorders. This technology is particularly promising for individuals with paralysis or motor neuron diseases. "Brain-computer interfaces can offer a new communication and control channel for those with severe motor disabilities," states Dr. Leigh Hochberg, a neurologist and engineer working on BCIs (Hochberg, 2012).

Exploring MMIs as a biohack involves pushing the boundaries of human cognition and exploring the interface between biology and technology. It embodies a futuristic approach to enhancing and augmenting human capabilities, blurring the lines between the human mind and machines. This cutting-edge field of biohacking promises to unlock new frontiers in human potential and capability.

Isochronic Tones for Focus: Use auditory stimuli to enhance concentration.

Isochronic Tones for Focus, a technique gaining popularity in the biohacking community, involves listening to specific auditory stimuli to enhance concentration and mental clarity. Isochronic tones are single tones that are turned on and off rapidly, creating distinct pulses of sound. This method is believed to influence brainwave patterns and can be used to foster a state of deep focus. Dr. Gerald Oster, known for his research in auditory and neurological science, explains, "Isochronic tones can help synchronize brainwave frequencies, which can positively affect cognitive functions like focus and concentration" (Oster, 1973). His research underlines the potential of auditory stimuli in brainwave entrainment.

Unlike binaural beats, isochronic tones do not require stereo headphones and are effective even when played over speakers. These tones work by creating a pattern of sound that the brain naturally syncs with, potentially leading to enhanced mental performance. "Using isochronic tones can be a powerful way to boost productivity and focus, especially in those with attention difficulties," states Dr. Tina Huang, a neuroscientist who has studied the effects of sound on brain function (Huang, 2007).

Incorporating isochronic tones into a daily routine can be a simple yet effective biohack for improving focus and attention. Whether used during work, study, or meditation, these auditory stimuli offer a non-invasive method to potentially enhance cognitive performance and mental clarity. This approach exemplifies the biohacking ethos of using scientifically grounded techniques to optimize the body and mind's capabilities.

Myofascial Release Techniques: Use tools like foam rollers for muscle recovery.

Myofascial Release Techniques, increasingly adopted within the biohacking community, involve using tools like foam rollers, lacrosse balls, and massage sticks to relieve muscle tightness, improve mobility, and aid in recovery. This method targets the fascia, a connective tissue surrounding muscles, to reduce soreness and improve tissue health. Dr. Robert Schleip, a fascia researcher and director of the Fascia Research Group, explains, "Myofascial release can alleviate pain, increase range of motion, and enhance tissue recovery" (Schleip, 2012). Schleip's research highlights the importance of fascial health in overall muscular function.

Using tools like foam rollers applies pressure to specific points on the body, aiding in the breakdown of tight muscle knots and the release of the fascia. This self-myofascial release (SMR) can be particularly beneficial after intense exercise or prolonged periods of sitting. "Foam rolling can be an effective tool for reducing muscle soreness and improving post-workout recovery," states Dr. Mark A. Tarnopolsky, a professor of pediatrics and exercise science (Tarnopolsky, 2013).

Incorporating myofascial release techniques into a regular fitness or recovery routine is a practical biohack for managing muscle soreness and enhancing physical performance. This approach exemplifies the biohacking principle of utilizing simple, effective tools to maintain and improve bodily function and well-being.

Lucid Dream Training: Learn to control and benefit from your dreams.

Lucid Dream Training, a practice gaining momentum in the biohacking community, involves techniques to become conscious during dreams and exert some level of control over them. This skill allows individuals to explore and interact with their dream environment, potentially leading to unique insights and psychological benefits. Dr. Stephen LaBerge, a pioneer in lucid dreaming research, explains, "Lucid dreaming is a learnable skill that can provide opportunities for adventure, increased self-awareness, and problem-solving" (LaBerge, 1985). His research indicates the potential for lucid dreaming to enhance cognitive abilities and emotional well-being.

Techniques for inducing lucid dreams include maintaining a dream journal, performing reality checks throughout the day, and using specific mental techniques before sleep. These methods aim to increase self-awareness and mindfulness, which can carry over into the dream state. "Lucid dreaming can be a powerful tool for overcoming fears, resolving anxieties, and exploring one's inner self," says Dr. Clare Johnson, an expert in dream therapy (Johnson, 2017).

Adopting lucid dream training as a biohack offers a non-invasive and natural way to explore the subconscious mind, enhance creativity, and improve problem-solving skills. It represents a unique intersection of sleep science and personal development, aligning with the biohacking ethos of self-exploration and optimization.

Biometric Analysis: Regularly check vital metrics like blood pressure and blood sugar.

Biometric Analysis, a fundamental practice in the biohacking community, involves regularly monitoring vital metrics such as blood pressure, blood sugar, heart rate, and cholesterol levels. This proactive approach allows individuals to keep track of their health status and detect potential issues early on. Dr. Michael Snyder, a professor and leader in genomics and personalized medicine, emphasizes the importance of biometric monitoring: "Regular tracking of key biometrics can provide valuable insights into your health and help you make informed lifestyle decisions" (Snyder, 2015). Snyder's work advocates for the use of personal data in managing and optimizing health.

Monitoring blood pressure and blood sugar levels are particularly crucial for individuals at risk of hypertension and diabetes, respectively. Regular checks enable timely interventions and lifestyle adjustments. "Understanding your blood pressure and blood sugar levels is essential for preventing and managing cardiovascular diseases and diabetes," explains Dr. Ronald M. Krauss, a renowned expert in lipidology (Krauss, 2018).

Incorporating biometric analysis into daily routines represents a biohacking strategy focused on prevention and self-awareness. It exemplifies the principle of using data-driven methods to take control of one's health, encouraging proactive rather than reactive health management. This approach aligns with the broader biohacking ethos of optimizing health through informed, personalized strategies.

Dopamine Fasting: Temporarily abstain from pleasurable activities to reset your brain's reward system.

Dopamine Fasting, an emerging trend in the biohacking community, involves temporarily abstaining from activities that are highly stimulating or pleasurable, like social media, gaming, or even certain foods, to reset the brain's dopamine levels. This concept is based on the premise that reducing the overstimulation of dopamine receptors can help to regain control over impulsive behaviors and increase satisfaction from simpler pleasures. Dr. Cameron Sepah, a clinical psychologist who popularized dopamine fasting, explains, "Dopamine fasting is a way to regain control over your impulses by taking a break from overstimulating behaviors" (Sepah, 2019). His approach focuses on reducing the constant bombardment of stimuli that can lead to addictive patterns.

The practice of dopamine fasting doesn't imply that dopamine itself is bad, but rather that the constant and intense stimulation of dopamine pathways can lead to a desensitization, where more and more stimulation is needed to experience pleasure or motivation. By periodically stepping away from high-dopamine activities, individuals aim to reset their brain's reward system, leading to increased focus, productivity, and enjoyment in daily activities. "It's about resetting your neurochemical balance to appreciate everyday activities again," notes Dr. Sepah (Sepah, 2019).

Adopting dopamine fasting as a biohack involves identifying and taking breaks from behaviors that are excessively rewarding or stimulating. This practice aligns with the biohacking principle of self-experimentation and mindfulness, focusing on regaining balance in one's mental and emotional state. Dopamine fasting represents a strategic retreat from the constant engagement of modern life, offering a path to a more balanced, controlled, and satisfying life experience.

Cold Plunge Pools: Use brief, intense cold immersion for recovery and mental sharpness.

Cold Plunge Pools, a practice widely embraced in the biohacking community, involve immersing oneself in ice-cold water for brief periods. This intense cold exposure is used for recovery after intense physical activity and to enhance mental sharpness. Wim Hof, known for his cold endurance feats, advocates for cold immersion, stating, "Regular exposure to cold water has profound impacts on health, including reduced inflammation, improved sleep, and heightened mental clarity" (Hof, 2020). Hof's method, which combines breathing techniques with cold exposure, underscores the health benefits of this practice.

The physiological effects of immersing in cold water include constricted blood vessels, which flush out toxins and metabolic waste from the muscles, reducing soreness and speeding up recovery. Cold immersion also triggers a flood of endorphins, leading to improved mood and mental alertness. "Cold water immersion can act as a form of stress that, over time, strengthens the body's adaptive responses to stress," explains Dr. Rhonda Patrick, a biomedical scientist (Patrick, 2016).

Incorporating cold plunge pools into a wellness routine is a powerful biohack for enhancing physical and mental performance. This practice exemplifies the biohacking ethos of challenging the body to adapt and improve, aligning with a lifestyle focused on optimizing health and resilience. Cold immersion, while initially uncomfortable, offers a unique and invigorating way to boost recovery and mental acuity.

Hypoxic Training: Train in low oxygen conditions to increase endurance and performance.

Hypoxic Training, a method increasingly explored in the biohacking community, involves training in environments with reduced oxygen levels to enhance endurance and overall athletic performance. This practice simulates high-altitude conditions, prompting the body to adapt by increasing red blood cell production and improving oxygen efficiency. Dr. Benjamin Levine, a professor of exercise sciences, explains, "Training in hypoxia or low-oxygen environments can significantly improve cardiovascular and pulmonary efficiency, as well as increase stamina" (Levine, 2015). Levine's research indicates the potential benefits of hypoxic training for athletes and fitness enthusiasts.

Typically, hypoxic training is conducted using specialized equipment like hypoxic tents or masks that limit oxygen intake, mimicking the conditions found at high altitudes. This method is particularly popular among endurance athletes, as it can lead to improved performance at sea level. "Hypoxic training can give athletes a competitive edge by enhancing their body's ability to utilize oxygen more effectively," states Dr. Robert Chapman, an expert in sports performance (Chapman, 2014).

Adopting hypoxic training as a biohack involves carefully planned and monitored sessions to ensure safety and effectiveness. This approach exemplifies the biohacking principle of pushing the body's limits to adapt and improve, offering a cutting-edge strategy for those seeking to boost their physical capabilities and endurance. Hypoxic training represents a convergence of exercise science and environmental manipulation, harnessing the body's natural adaptive responses for peak performance.

Alkaline Water: Drink pH-balanced water for potential health benefits.

Alkaline Water, a concept embraced within the biohacking community, revolves around consuming water with a higher pH level than regular drinking water, with the belief that it can neutralize acid in the bloodstream, leading to potential health benefits. Advocates of alkaline water claim that it can improve hydration, increase energy, and slow aging processes. Dr. Jamie Koufman, a physician specializing in acid reflux, suggests, "Alkaline water can neutralize the acid in your bloodstream and help your body metabolize nutrients more effectively, leading to improved health and performance" (Koufman, 2012). Koufman's research indicates potential benefits of alkaline water in balancing the body's pH levels.

The idea behind alkaline water is that a more alkaline diet, including water with a higher pH, can help counteract the effects of an acidic diet, which is common in modern lifestyles. This shift is believed to aid in reducing acidity-related issues such as fatigue, poor digestion, and certain chronic diseases. "Drinking alkaline water may have benefits for those who suffer from acid reflux," notes Dr. Koufman (Koufman, 2012).

Incorporating alkaline water into a daily routine is a biohack aimed at optimizing bodily functions and health. It aligns with the principle of making small, incremental changes to improve overall well-being. While the scientific community is still evaluating the full range of benefits claimed by alkaline water proponents, it remains a popular choice among biohackers for its potential health-enhancing properties.

Biohacking Supplements for Gut Health: Use prebiotics, probiotics, and digestive enzymes.

Biohacking Supplements for Gut Health, an approach increasingly recognized in the biohacking community, involves using prebiotics, probiotics, and digestive enzymes to enhance gastrointestinal function and overall health. Prebiotics are dietary fibers that feed beneficial gut bacteria, while probiotics are live bacteria that add to the population of healthy microbes in the gut. Digestive enzymes, on the other hand, aid in breaking down food into nutrients the body can absorb. Dr. Michael Gershon, a professor of pathology and cell biology known for his work on gut health, states, "A healthy gut flora supported by prebiotics and probiotics plays a crucial role in digestion, immunity, and overall health" (Gershon, 2018). Gershon's insights highlight the interconnectedness of gut health with broader bodily functions.

The rationale behind using these supplements is to create a more favorable gut environment, which can lead to improved digestion, stronger immune function, and even mood regulation. "Probiotics can help restore the natural balance of gut bacteria, leading to improved gut health and, consequently, overall well-being," says Dr. Alessio Fasano, a gastroenterologist and researcher in gut health (Fasano, 2014).

Incorporating these gut health supplements into a daily health regimen represents a biohacking strategy focused on nurturing the gut microbiome, which is increasingly recognized as a key factor in overall health. This approach exemplifies the biohacking ethos of using scientific knowledge and self-experimentation to optimize the body's functioning and promote health and wellness.

Glycemic Index Management: Focus on low-glycemic foods for stable blood sugar.

Glycemic Index Management, a dietary approach gaining traction in the biohacking community, focuses on consuming low-glycemic foods to maintain stable blood sugar levels. The glycemic index (GI) measures how quickly foods cause increases in blood sugar levels. Low-GI foods, such as most vegetables, whole grains, and legumes, are digested and absorbed more slowly, leading to a gradual rise in blood sugar. Dr. David Jenkins, the creator of the glycemic index, explains, "Foods with a low glycemic index provide a more stable blood sugar and sustain energy levels longer, which can be beneficial for weight management and overall health" (Jenkins, 1981). Jenkins' work underscores the importance of GI in dietary choices.

By focusing on low-GI foods, individuals can avoid spikes in blood sugar, which can lead to improved insulin sensitivity and reduced risk of type 2 diabetes. "Managing glycemic load is not only important for diabetics but also for anyone seeking to maintain steady energy levels and reduce hunger cravings," states Dr. Walter Willett, a professor of epidemiology and nutrition (Willett, 2002).

Adopting a low-glycemic diet as part of a biohacking strategy involves choosing foods that support stable blood glucose levels, which can lead to better energy management, mood stability, and overall metabolic health. This approach aligns with the biohacking principle of making informed, data-driven dietary choices to optimize physical health and well-being.

Autophagy Induction Fasting: Fast to promote cellular cleanup and rejuvenation.

Autophagy Induction Fasting, an approach widely recognized and practiced in the biohacking community, involves fasting to activate the body's autophagy process, a natural mechanism of the cell that removes unnecessary or dysfunctional components. Autophagy, which literally means 'self-eating,' is a cellular cleanup process where cells break down and recycle damaged proteins and organelles. Dr. Yoshinori Ohsumi, a Nobel laureate for his work on autophagy, explains, "Fasting activates autophagy, which helps slow down the aging process and has a positive impact on cell renewal" (Ohsumi, 2016). His research has been pivotal in understanding how fasting can induce autophagy, leading to cellular rejuvenation and health benefits.

Fasting to induce autophagy can take various forms, including intermittent fasting or more extended fasts. During periods of fasting, when energy intake is low, the body increases autophagy, promoting cellular repair and regeneration. This process is believed to play a role in preventing a range of diseases, including cancer, neurodegenerative disorders, and infections. "Autophagy is an essential, homeostatic process that protects against diseases of aging," states Dr. Beth Levine, a researcher in autophagy (Levine, 2017).

Adopting autophagy induction fasting as a biohack involves strategically timed fasting periods to promote the body's natural self-cleansing process. This practice aligns with the biohacking ethos of utilizing the body's intrinsic mechanisms to optimize health and longevity. Autophagy induction fasting represents a proactive approach to health maintenance, leveraging the body's own tools for cellular maintenance and rejuvenation.

Transcranial Direct Current Stimulation (tDCS): Use mild electrical currents for cognitive enhancement.

Transcranial Direct Current Stimulation (tDCS), a neurostimulation technique embraced by the biohacking community, involves applying mild electrical currents to the scalp to enhance cognitive functions. This non-invasive method is used to stimulate specific areas of the brain, with the goal of improving attention, problem-solving abilities, and memory. Dr. Michael Nitsche, a pioneer in tDCS research, notes, "tDCS can modulate neuronal activity, which in turn has the potential to enhance cognitive performance, particularly in learning and memory tasks" (Nitsche, 2008). His research has demonstrated the efficacy of tDCS in cognitive enhancement.

tDCS devices pass a low electrical current (usually 1-2 milliamperes) through electrodes placed on the head. This current is thought to increase neuronal excitability in the targeted brain regions, making it easier for neurons to fire. The technique has gained popularity among those seeking to boost their cognitive abilities, whether for professional development, academic purposes, or personal interest. "tDCS is being explored as a tool not only for cognitive enhancement but also for potential therapeutic applications in various neurological conditions," explains Dr. Marom Bikson, a biomedical engineer specializing in neuromodulation (Bikson, 2012).

Incorporating tDCS into a cognitive enhancement regimen represents a biohacking strategy focused on leveraging neuroscience for personal development. This approach is aligned with the biohacking principle of using technology to optimize the human brain's capabilities, offering a novel way to enhance mental function and cognitive health.

UVB Lamp Exposure: For vitamin D synthesis in low-sunlight environments.

UVB Lamp Exposure, a method increasingly utilized in the biohacking community, involves the use of ultraviolet B (UVB) lamps to stimulate vitamin D synthesis, especially in environments with low sunlight. This approach is particularly beneficial during winter months or for individuals living in higher latitudes where natural sun exposure is limited. Dr. Michael Holick, a professor of medicine and a leading expert in vitamin D research, states, "UVB lamp exposure can be an effective way to maintain adequate vitamin D levels when natural sunlight is scarce" (Holick, 2007). Holick's research emphasizes the importance of vitamin D for bone health, immune function, and overall well-being.

Vitamin D, often referred to as the "sunshine vitamin," is produced in the skin in response to UVB light. Adequate levels of vitamin D are crucial for calcium absorption, bone health, and immune system function. Inadequate vitamin D levels can lead to a range of health issues, including bone disorders, cardiovascular diseases, and weakened immune response. "Using a UVB lamp for short, controlled periods can help boost vitamin D levels, mimicking the natural process that occurs in the skin during sun exposure," explains Dr. Holick (Holick, 2007).

Incorporating UVB lamp exposure into a health routine is a biohacking strategy aimed at countering the lack of natural sunlight in certain environments. It exemplifies the biohacking ethos of adapting to environmental limitations to optimize health, providing a practical solution to maintain essential vitamin levels for overall health and disease prevention.

Carbon 60 Supplements: Investigate the potential longevity benefits of C60.

Carbon 60 Supplements, often referred to as C60, have garnered interest in the biohacking community for their potential longevity and health benefits. C60 is a molecule composed of 60 carbon atoms forming a hollow spherical structure, resembling a soccer ball. Its unique structure has prompted research into its antioxidant properties and potential health benefits. Dr. Fathi Moussa, a pharmacologist who led a seminal study on C60, notes, "C60 has a high affinity for both electrons and protons, which suggests it has powerful antioxidant properties" (Moussa, 2012). His study, which showed extended lifespan in rats treated with C60, sparked interest in its potential for human longevity.

The hypothesis is that C60 can scavenge free radicals, thereby reducing oxidative stress, a major contributor to aging and many chronic diseases. Proponents of C60 supplements suggest that they can improve cellular function, reduce inflammation, and extend lifespan. "The antioxidant capacity of C60 might be harnessed to protect cells from aging and damage," explains Dr. Moussa (Moussa, 2012).

While the research on C60 is still in its early stages, particularly regarding its effects on human health, it represents an intriguing area of exploration within biohacking for those interested in anti-aging and longevity. C60 supplements exemplify the biohacking community's interest in exploring novel substances that have the potential to enhance health and extend lifespan.

Quantum Meditation: Explore advanced meditation techniques for deeper relaxation.

Quantum Meditation, an advanced technique gaining traction in the biohacking community, delves into deeper states of relaxation and consciousness exploration. This method combines traditional meditation principles with concepts of quantum physics, focusing on the connection between mind and matter. Dr. John Hagelin, a quantum physicist and advocate for integrative meditation techniques, explains, "Quantum meditation allows individuals to tap into deeper levels of awareness, aligning thoughts and consciousness with the fundamental dynamics of the universe" (Hagelin, 2014). His research posits that such practices can lead to profound mental clarity and well-being.

This form of meditation often involves visualization techniques and focused intention, aiming to influence one's reality at a quantum level. Practitioners believe that by aligning their thoughts and energy with desired outcomes, they can manifest changes in their physical and mental states. "The practice of quantum meditation can create a powerful shift in one's perception and experience of reality," notes Dr. Hagelin (Hagelin, 2014).

Adopting quantum meditation as a biohack involves exploring the interplay between consciousness and the physical world, pushing the boundaries of traditional meditation practices. This approach aligns with the biohacking ethos of self-experimentation and exploration, aiming to harness the mind's potential to affect personal health and reality. Quantum meditation represents an advanced, holistic approach to well-being, emphasizing the profound impact of mental states on overall life experience.

Chronobiology Adjustments: Align activities with your biological clock for optimal performance.

Chronobiology Adjustments, a concept embraced by the biohacking community, involves aligning daily activities with the body's natural circadian rhythms to optimize performance, health, and well-being. Chronobiology is the science of biological rhythms, including the circadian rhythm, which is the body's internal clock that regulates sleep-wake cycles and other physiological processes. Dr. Till Roenneberg, a professor of chronobiology, states, "Living in sync with your internal clock and respecting your individual chronotype can significantly improve health and performance" (Roenneberg, 2012). Roenneberg's research emphasizes the importance of aligning lifestyle habits with our biological rhythms.

This approach includes adjusting sleep patterns, meal times, and periods of work or exercise according to one's natural circadian rhythm. For instance, understanding whether one is a 'morning person' or 'night owl' can guide the scheduling of challenging tasks or workouts at times when one is most alert and energetic. "Aligning your schedule with your circadian rhythm can lead to more effective sleep, improved cognitive function, and overall better health," explains Dr. Phyllis Zee, a sleep medicine specialist (Zee, 2017).

Incorporating chronobiology adjustments into daily life is a biohacking strategy that focuses on the synchronization of external schedules with internal biological clocks. This method exemplifies the biohacking principle of using scientific understanding of the body to improve daily functioning and wellness. Chronobiology adjustments represent a proactive approach to enhancing life quality through the optimization of biological rhythms.

Nasal Breathing Exercises: Improve breathing efficiency and lung function.

Nasal Breathing Exercises, increasingly recognized in the biohacking community, focus on enhancing breathing efficiency and lung function by emphasizing inhalation and exhalation through the nose. This practice is based on the principle that nasal breathing is more beneficial than mouth breathing, as it offers better filtration of impurities, regulates air temperature, and optimizes oxygen uptake. Dr. John Douillard, a proponent of nasal breathing and author on body-mind health, explains, "Nasal breathing drives deeper diaphragmatic activation, improving lung function, increasing oxygenation, and reducing stress" (Douillard, 2016). His work highlights the physiological benefits of this breathing method.

Nasal breathing exercises involve techniques to train the body to breathe more efficiently through the nose, even during physical activities or sleep. These exercises can lead to improved endurance, better sleep quality, and enhanced mental clarity. "Practicing nasal breathing can significantly impact overall health, from improving cardiovascular function to enhancing athletic performance," states Dr. Douillard (Douillard, 2016).

Incorporating nasal breathing exercises into daily routines is a biohack that aligns with the principle of optimizing the body's natural functions. This approach exemplifies a simple yet effective method to improve respiratory health, stress management, and physical endurance. Nasal breathing exercises represent a practical and accessible tool for anyone looking to enhance their breathing efficiency and overall well-being.

Barefoot Running: Adapt to natural running to improve posture and reduce injuries.

Barefoot Running, a practice gaining popularity in the biohacking community, emphasizes running without shoes or with minimal footwear to adapt to a more natural running form. This approach is based on the belief that barefoot running encourages a forefoot or midfoot strike, which is thought to be more natural and less impactful than the heel strike commonly seen in shod runners. Dr. Daniel Lieberman, a professor of human evolutionary biology, explains, "Barefoot running can lead to a more natural gait, potentially reducing the risk of common running injuries" (Lieberman, 2010). Lieberman's research suggests that barefoot running can improve foot biomechanics and posture.

Advocates of barefoot running argue that it strengthens the muscles, tendons, and ligaments of the foot, leading to improved balance and posture. Running without the cushioning of modern shoes is believed to enhance sensory feedback from the feet to the brain, promoting a more responsive running style. "Adapting to barefoot running requires a transition period, but it can lead to improvements in foot strength and overall running mechanics," notes Dr. Lieberman (Lieberman, 2010).

Incorporating barefoot running into a fitness routine is a biohack that aligns with the principle of returning to natural, evolutionary-based practices for health and performance. This approach exemplifies a shift towards more holistic and integrative methods in physical training, focusing on injury prevention and the optimization of natural body movements. Barefoot running represents a reconnection with natural human biomechanics, offering a potential path to improved running efficiency and reduced injury risk.

Neuro-linguistic Programming (NLP): Use NLP for personal development and mental health.

Neuro-linguistic Programming (NLP), a technique embraced by the biohacking community, involves the use of language and communication strategies to influence thought patterns and behaviors for personal development and improved mental health. NLP is based on the premise that there is a connection between neurological processes, language, and behavioral patterns learned through experience, and that these can be changed to achieve specific goals in life. Dr. Richard Bandler, a co-creator of NLP, explains, "NLP provides tools and techniques to reprogram your mind, enhancing communication, personal growth, and emotional well-being" (Bandler, 1980). His work highlights the potential of NLP in personal development and therapy.

NLP techniques include visualization, reframing, and the use of specific language patterns to influence one's subconscious mind. Practitioners believe that by changing how one perceives events and interacts with the world, it is possible to alter emotional and behavioral responses. "NLP can be particularly effective in overcoming fears, phobias, and limiting beliefs, leading to improved confidence and decision-making," states Dr. Bandler (Bandler, 1980).

Adopting NLP as a biohack involves exploring and modifying the linguistic and cognitive processes to improve communication, emotional health, and overall life satisfaction. This approach aligns with the biohacking ethos of self-improvement and optimization, offering a method for enhancing mental and emotional well-being through the strategic use of language and thought. NLP represents a tool for personal transformation, grounded in the understanding of the psychological and linguistic influences on behavior and experience.

Dynamic Neurofeedback: Use advanced feedback for brain training and relaxation.

Dynamic Neurofeedback, a sophisticated technique in the realm of biohacking, utilizes advanced feedback systems to train the brain, enhancing relaxation and cognitive performance. This method involves monitoring brainwave activity in real-time and providing instant feedback, enabling individuals to learn how to modulate their mental states. Dr. Valdeane Brown, a developer of advanced neurofeedback systems, explains, "Dynamic neurofeedback offers a way for the brain to reorganize itself. It's like holding up a mirror to the mind, allowing it to adjust its own patterns for better function" (Brown, 2015). Brown's research underscores the potential of neurofeedback in self-regulation and brain optimization.

During dynamic neurofeedback sessions, sensors placed on the scalp measure electrical activity in the brain. This information is then reflected back through visual or auditory signals. The brain uses this feedback to recognize its patterns and make adjustments, leading to enhanced relaxation, focus, and mental agility. "This form of neurofeedback can be particularly effective for stress reduction, improving attention, and overcoming sleep issues," notes Dr. Brown (Brown, 2015).

Incorporating dynamic neurofeedback into a mental wellness routine is a biohack that aligns with the principle of using technology to optimize brain function. This approach represents a fusion of neuroscience and self-improvement, offering a sophisticated method for enhancing brain health and overall cognitive abilities. Dynamic neurofeedback provides a non-invasive, drug-free option for those seeking to improve their mental capabilities and resilience.

Isochronic Tones for Sleep: Utilize sound waves to enhance sleep quality.

Isochronic Tones for Sleep, a technique increasingly utilized in the biohacking community, involves the use of sound waves set at specific frequencies to enhance the quality of sleep. Isochronic tones work by emitting a single tone that is manually turned on and off at regular intervals, creating a distinct pulsing rhythm. This method is thought to influence brainwave patterns, promoting relaxation and sleep. Dr. Helane Wahbeh, a researcher in mind-body medicine, explains, "Isochronic tones can entrain brain waves to slower frequencies that are conducive to relaxation and sleep" (Wahbeh, 2007). Her research indicates the potential of isochronic tones in aiding sleep disorders.

These tones are designed to guide the brain into a state of deep relaxation, progressing toward the slow brainwave patterns characteristic of deep sleep. "Listening to isochronic tones before bed can help individuals who struggle with falling asleep or maintaining deep sleep," notes Dr. Wahbeh (Wahbeh, 2007).

Using isochronic tones for sleep enhancement is a biohacking strategy that combines technology and neuroscience. By entraining brainwaves to a specific frequency, isochronic tones offer a non-invasive method to improve sleep quality, which is crucial for overall health and well-being. This approach exemplifies the biohacking ethos of leveraging scientific knowledge and tools to optimize the body's natural functions.

Sirtuin-Activating Compounds (SACs): Investigate the potential of SACs in promoting longevity and health.

Sirtuin-Activating Compounds (SACs), a subject of growing interest in the biohacking community, involve the use of specific compounds that activate sirtuins, a group of proteins believed to play a key role in aging and cellular health. Sirtuins are known to influence aging, gene expression, and the body's response to stress. Dr. David

Sinclair, a professor of genetics well-known for his research on aging, emphasizes the potential of SACs, stating, "Sirtuin-activating compounds have shown promise in promoting longevity and improving healthspan by mimicking the effects of caloric restriction" (Sinclair, 2013). His work suggests that SACs could be instrumental in the fight against aging and age-related diseases.

One of the most well-known SACs is resveratrol, a compound found in red wine and grapes, which has been shown to activate sirtuins and mimic the beneficial effects of caloric restriction without the need to reduce food intake. Other compounds being investigated include SIRT1-activating compounds (STACs) and NAD+ precursors, both of which are believed to influence sirtuin activity positively. "Sirtuins are important for maintaining cellular health and resilience, and activating them could have significant health benefits," notes Dr. Sinclair (Sinclair, 2013).

Investigating and utilizing SACs as a biohack involves exploring these compounds' potential to enhance longevity and overall health. This approach aligns with the biohacking community's goal of extending healthspan and improving the quality of life through scientific advancements and lifestyle interventions. SACs represent a cutting-edge frontier in biohacking, focusing on cellular mechanisms that could unlock the secrets to longer, healthier lives.

Pulsed Electromagnetic Field Therapy (PEMF): Use electromagnetic fields to improve cellular function.

Pulsed Electromagnetic Field Therapy (PEMF), a method increasingly adopted in the biohacking community, involves the use of electromagnetic fields to stimulate and enhance cellular function and overall health. PEMF therapy employs electromagnetic waves at various frequencies to interact with the body's natural magnetic field, promoting healing and cellular repair. Dr. William Pawluk, a former Johns Hopkins University physician and a leading authority on PEMF, explains, "PEMF works at a cellular level, boosting cell metabolism and enhancing the body's natural ability to heal itself" (Pawluk, 2015). Pawluk's insights underline the potential of PEMF in supporting the body's intrinsic healing processes.

The application of PEMF therapy can range from pain management and injury recovery to enhancing overall energy levels. The electromagnetic fields generated by PEMF devices are thought to stimulate the electrical charges around and within cells, improving cellular function and health. "PEMF therapy has been shown to be effective in reducing pain and inflammation, accelerating bone and tissue repair, and improving circulation," states Dr. Pawluk (Pawluk, 2015).

Incorporating PEMF into a health and wellness routine is a biohack that utilizes advanced technology to optimize the body's natural healing capabilities. This approach is aligned with the biohacking principle of using scientifically grounded methods to enhance physical and mental well-being. PEMF therapy represents a non-invasive, innovative approach to health maintenance and recovery, offering a promising tool for those seeking to improve their overall health and quality of life.

Virtual Reality for Pain Management: Utilize VR environments to manage and reduce pain perception.

Virtual Reality for Pain Management, a novel approach in the biohacking community, involves using VR environments as a tool to manage and reduce pain perception. This technique leverages the immersive and distracting qualities of virtual reality to draw a user's attention away from pain, effectively altering the perception of pain. Dr. Hunter Hoffman, a leading researcher in VR pain management, notes, "Virtual reality can be more effective than traditional pain management techniques because it immersively distracts the patient, reducing their perception of pain" (Hoffman, 2016). His research indicates the significant potential of VR in pain therapy.

In VR pain management, individuals wear VR headsets that transport them to digitally created environments, which can range from serene landscapes to engaging interactive scenarios. These immersive experiences are designed to occupy the mind so fully that it processes less pain signals. "The immersive quality of VR can create a form of analgesia by occupying the brain's attention capacity, offering a promising alternative for pain relief," explains Dr. Hoffman (Hoffman, 2016).

Adopting VR for pain management represents a biohacking strategy that combines technology and psychology to address physical discomfort. This approach is especially beneficial for those seeking non-pharmacological options for pain relief. VR for pain management exemplifies the innovative use of technology in healthcare, offering an effective and engaging way to manage pain and improve the quality of life for individuals suffering from chronic pain or undergoing medical procedures.

Smart Pill Technology: Track digestion and nutrient absorption with ingestible sensors.

Smart Pill Technology, an emerging trend in the biohacking community, involves using ingestible sensors to track digestive processes and nutrient absorption. These advanced technological capsules provide real-time data on various aspects of the gastrointestinal system. Dr. Giovanni Traverso, a gastroenterologist and biomedical engineer at Brigham and Women's Hospital, explains, "Smart pills can revolutionize the way we monitor and understand the gut's health, providing valuable insights into digestion, absorption, and gut microbiome" (Traverso, 2017). His work underscores the potential of these devices in personal health monitoring and diagnostics.

Once ingested, these smart pills can measure factors such as pH levels, temperature, and pressure within the gastrointestinal tract. Some are even capable of capturing images, offering a detailed view of the intestinal lining. This data can be crucial for diagnosing conditions like Crohn's disease, ulcers, and irritable bowel syndrome. "The ability to track the internal workings of the digestive system can lead to more personalized and effective treatments for gastrointestinal disorders," notes Dr. Traverso (Traverso, 2017).

Incorporating Smart Pill Technology into health management is a biohack that leverages cutting-edge advancements in medical science. It aligns with the principle of using data-driven approaches for health optimization and personalized medicine. This technology represents a significant leap forward in the biohacking community, providing a non-invasive, comprehensive tool for understanding and improving digestive health.

Whole Body Vibration Training: Use vibration platforms for improved muscle strength and bone density.

Whole Body Vibration Training, a method adopted by the biohacking community, involves using vibration platforms that transmit energy to the body, causing muscles to contract and relax multiple times per second. This form of training is touted for its benefits in improving muscle strength, bone density, and overall fitness. Dr. Carmelo Bosco, an exercise physiologist who conducted early research on vibration training, notes, "Whole body vibration can enhance muscle strength and performance, potentially more efficiently than conventional exercise" (Bosco, 1999). His research suggests significant gains in strength and power from this training method.

These platforms work by generating vibrations that stimulate muscle fibers, leading to improved muscle activation compared to traditional exercises. The vibrations also stimulate bone cells, which can help improve bone density, making it a beneficial tool for combating osteoporosis. "Vibration training has shown promise in improving balance, muscle strength, and bone density, especially in older adults," states Dr. Bosco (Bosco, 1999).

Incorporating whole body vibration training into a fitness routine is a biohack that utilizes advanced technology to enhance physical conditioning. This approach aligns with the biohacking ethos of finding efficient and effective methods to improve health and performance. Whole body vibration training represents a unique and innovative way to enhance physical fitness, offering a time-efficient solution for improving muscle strength and bone health.

Optogenetics: Experiment with light to control cells in the brain for mood regulation.

Optogenetics, a groundbreaking technique in neuroscience and biohacking, involves the use of light to control cells in the brain, particularly for mood regulation and understanding brain functions. This method combines genetic engineering with light to control individual neurons' activity, offering precise control over brain circuits. Dr. Karl Deisseroth, a pioneer in the development of optogenetics, explains, "Optogenetics allows us to understand the complex patterns of neural activity that underlie behavior, emotions, and thought processes" (Deisseroth, 2010). His research highlights the potential of optogenetics in unraveling the mysteries of the brain.

In optogenetics, light-sensitive proteins are introduced into specific neurons in the brain. When these neurons are exposed to light of certain wavelengths, they can be activated or inhibited, allowing researchers to study the effects of these changes on behavior and mood. "This technique can be used to dissect the neural mechanisms underlying mood disorders and potentially develop new treatments," states Dr. Deisseroth (Deisseroth, 2010).

Using optogenetics as a biohack involves a deep exploration of brain function and mood regulation, representing a fusion of biology, technology, and neuroscience. This approach is particularly exciting for its potential to develop new treatments for neurological and psychiatric disorders. Optogenetics embodies the cutting-edge of biohacking, offering a window into the complex workings of the brain and a powerful tool for understanding and potentially manipulating brain function for better health and well-being.

Molecular Hydrogen Inhalation: Explore the therapeutic benefits of hydrogen gas on oxidative stress.

Molecular Hydrogen Inhalation, a practice gaining attention in the biohacking community, involves inhaling hydrogen gas to explore its therapeutic benefits, particularly against oxidative stress. Molecular hydrogen (H2) is a colorless, odorless gas that has been studied for its antioxidant properties. Dr. Shigeo Ohta, a prominent researcher in the field, explains, "Molecular hydrogen acts as a selective antioxidant, reducing cytotoxic oxygen radicals and protecting cells from oxidative stress" (Ohta, 2007). His research suggests potential health benefits from hydrogen inhalation, particularly in reducing oxidative damage.

When inhaled, molecular hydrogen is thought to rapidly diffuse into tissues and cells, neutralizing harmful free radicals and reducing oxidative stress, which is linked to inflammation and various chronic diseases. "Inhaling hydrogen gas can provide therapeutic benefits for diseases where oxidative stress plays a significant role," states Dr. Ohta (Ohta, 2007).

Incorporating molecular hydrogen inhalation into a wellness routine represents a biohack that leverages the subtle yet powerful properties of this element. This approach aligns with the biohacking ethos of exploring novel and scientifically-backed methods to enhance health and combat the effects of aging. Molecular hydrogen inhalation is gaining traction as a non-invasive and innovative way to potentially protect the body against oxidative stress and promote overall well-being.

Artificial Intelligence Personal Health Assistants: Use AI for personalized health advice and tracking.

Artificial Intelligence (AI) Personal Health Assistants, a rapidly evolving tool in the biohacking community, leverage AI technology to provide personalized health advice and tracking. These digital assistants use algorithms to analyze health data, offer recommendations, and even predict potential health issues. Dr. Eric Topol, a cardiologist and digital medicine researcher, states, "AI personal health assistants have the potential to transform healthcare by offering customized guidance and monitoring based on individual health data" (Topol, 2019). Topol's insights underscore the potential of AI in personalizing healthcare and wellness strategies.

These AI-driven platforms can track a wide range of health metrics, from sleep patterns and physical activity to heart rate and blood glucose levels. By processing this data, AI health assistants can identify trends, offer insights into health habits, and suggest lifestyle changes. "The use of AI in personal health management can lead to more proactive and preventive healthcare, tailored to the individual's specific needs," explains Dr. Topol (Topol, 2019).

Incorporating AI personal health assistants into a health regimen represents a biohack that combines technology and data analytics for optimized health management. This approach exemplifies the biohacking principle of leveraging advanced technology to enhance understanding and control over one's health, offering a sophisticated, personalized approach to health tracking and management. AI personal health assistants represent a significant advancement in the integration of technology into personal wellness, providing accessible, data-driven insights for health optimization.

Chronic Inflammation Monitoring: Regularly test for markers of inflammation to prevent chronic diseases.

Chronic Inflammation Monitoring, a practice gaining importance in the biohacking community, involves regularly testing for markers of inflammation in the body to prevent and manage chronic diseases. Chronic inflammation is linked to a wide range of health issues, including heart disease, diabetes, and autoimmune disorders. Dr. Peter Libby, a cardiovascular medicine specialist, emphasizes, "Monitoring inflammation markers can be key in predicting and preventing various chronic diseases" (Libby, 2016). His research highlights the role of inflammation in many chronic health conditions.

Regular testing can include blood tests for markers like C-reactive protein (CRP), erythrocyte sedimentation rate (ESR), and specific interleukins, which can indicate the presence and level of inflammation in the body. "By keeping track of these inflammation markers, individuals can take early action to reduce risk factors and mitigate potential health issues," states Dr. Libby (Libby, 2016).

Incorporating chronic inflammation monitoring into a health maintenance routine is a biohack that aligns with a proactive approach to health. It exemplifies the principle of using data-driven strategies to preemptively address health issues. Regular monitoring of inflammation markers represents a practical approach to staying ahead of chronic diseases, offering valuable insights for personalized health interventions and lifestyle modifications.

Biohacking Skincare: Utilize advanced skincare routines based on genetic analysis.

Biohacking Skincare, an innovative approach in the realm of personal care and biohacking, involves tailoring advanced skincare routines based on individual genetic analysis. This method goes beyond traditional skincare by considering genetic factors that influence skin health, such as predisposition to certain skin conditions, elasticity, and aging. Dr. Rajani Katta, a dermatologist specializing in the link between nutrition and skin health, notes, "Genetic analysis can provide valuable insights into your skin's unique needs, allowing for more targeted and effective skincare" (Katta, 2018). Katta's approach highlights the importance of personalized skincare based on genetic makeup.

Genetic testing in skincare analyzes various genetic markers to inform decisions about skincare products and routines. This can include choosing products that target specific concerns like collagen production, moisture retention, or antioxidant protection. "Understanding your genetic predisposition can help in choosing skincare products that are more beneficial for your skin type and concerns," explains Dr. Katta (Katta, 2018).

Adopting biohacking skincare routines is a strategy that leverages the latest advancements in genetics and dermatology. This approach exemplifies the biohacking ethos of using scientific knowledge and technology to optimize personal health and well-being. Biohacking skincare represents a shift towards more personalized and effective skincare, aligning with the broader trend of personalized medicine and self-care.

Selective Androgen Receptor Modulators (SARMs): Investigate SARMs for muscle and bone health.

Selective Androgen Receptor Modulators (SARMs), a topic of interest within the biohacking community, involve the use of compounds that selectively target androgen receptors in the body, particularly in muscle and bone tissue. SARMs are being investigated for their potential to increase muscle mass, reduce fat, and strengthen bones without the side effects typically associated with anabolic steroids. Dr. James Dalton, a leading researcher in the development of SARMs, explains, "SARMs can selectively stimulate muscle and bone growth, showing promise for the treatment of muscle wasting diseases and osteoporosis" (Dalton, 2011). His research underscores the therapeutic potential of SARMs in muscle and bone health.

SARMs are designed to mimic the effects of testosterone by binding to androgen receptors, but with a more targeted approach that focuses on muscle and bone tissue. This specificity is believed to reduce the likelihood of side effects that are common with steroids, such as hormonal imbalances. "The selective action of SARMs could offer a safer alternative to traditional anabolic agents, particularly for muscle and bone-related conditions," states Dr. Dalton (Dalton, 2011).

Investigating and potentially using SARMs as a biohack involves exploring their role in enhancing physical performance, muscle building, and bone health. This approach is aligned with the biohacking principle of leveraging scientific advancements for personal health optimization. While SARMs present a promising frontier in muscle and bone therapeutics, their use requires careful consideration of legal and health implications. SARMs research represents a significant step towards developing safer and more effective treatments for muscle and bone-related conditions.

Anti-Aging Telomere Therapy: Focus on telomere lengthening for longevity.

Anti-Aging Telomere Therapy, a cutting-edge approach in the realm of biohacking, focuses on lengthening telomeres, the protective caps at the ends of chromosomes, as a strategy for promoting longevity and combating aging. Telomeres shorten as cells divide over time, and their length is considered a marker of biological aging. Dr. Elizabeth Blackburn, a Nobel laureate for her work on telomeres, notes, "Maintaining telomere length is thought to protect against age-related diseases and possibly extend lifespan" (Blackburn, 2009). Blackburn's research highlights the critical role of telomeres in cellular aging and longevity.

This approach to anti-aging involves strategies that may support or enhance telomere length, such as lifestyle changes, specific supplements, and emerging genetic therapies. Lifestyle factors like diet, exercise, and stress management have been shown to influence telomere length. Additionally, research into compounds like telomerase activators is ongoing, with the hope that they could directly impact telomere length. "The future of anti-aging therapy may lie in treatments that target telomeres, potentially slowing the aging process at a cellular level," suggests Dr. Blackburn (Blackburn, 2009).

Adopting anti-aging telomere therapy as a biohack involves a deep dive into the latest research and advancements in longevity science. This approach aligns with the biohacking ethos of using scientific understanding and innovative methods to extend healthspan and improve the quality of life. Anti-aging telomere therapy represents a frontier in biohacking, focusing on the cellular mechanisms of aging and seeking ways to preserve and enhance cellular health for longevity.

Cognitive Behavioral Therapy (CBT) for Sleep: Implement CBT techniques to improve sleep disorders.

Cognitive Behavioral Therapy (CBT) for Sleep, a method widely recognized and utilized in the biohacking community, involves applying CBT techniques to address and improve sleep disorders. CBT for sleep, often referred to as CBT-I (Cognitive Behavioral Therapy for Insomnia), is a structured program that helps individuals modify behaviors and thoughts that negatively impact sleep. Dr. Gregg D. Jacobs, an assistant professor of psychiatry and a sleep medicine specialist, explains, "CBT-I addresses the underlying causes of insomnia and has been shown to be a highly effective treatment for chronic sleep problems" (Jacobs, 2004). Jacobs' work emphasizes the effectiveness of CBT-I in improving sleep quality and duration.

CBT-I techniques include sleep restriction therapy, which limits the time spent in bed to match the actual sleep time, thus improving sleep efficiency. Another technique, stimulus control, helps break the association between the bedroom environment and wakefulness. "CBT-I also focuses on changing beliefs and attitudes about sleep, which can perpetuate sleep issues," notes Dr. Jacobs (Jacobs, 2004).

Incorporating CBT techniques for sleep improvement represents a biohack that focuses on cognitive and behavioral modification to enhance sleep quality. This approach aligns with the biohacking principle of using evidence-based strategies to improve health and well-being. CBT-I offers a non-pharmacological and effective method to tackle sleep disorders, emphasizing the power of mindset and behavior in achieving better sleep and, consequently, better overall health.

Nutrigenomic Analysis for Allergies: Customize diet plans based on genetic allergy profiles.

Nutrigenomic Analysis for Allergies, an approach gaining traction in the biohacking community, involves using genetic testing to understand individual allergic responses and customize diet plans accordingly. Nutrigenomics explores the relationship between genes, nutrition, and health, including how genetic variations can affect the way individuals react to different foods. Dr. Ahmed El-Sohemy, a professor of nutritional sciences, explains, "Nutrigenomic analysis can identify genetic predispositions to food allergies or intolerances, enabling personalized dietary recommendations for better health management" (El-Sohemy, 2015). His research underscores the potential of nutrigenomics in developing personalized nutrition strategies.

This type of analysis examines specific DNA markers related to immune responses and metabolic processes that can influence allergic reactions to foods. By identifying these genetic factors, individuals can tailor their diets to avoid triggering allergic responses or exacerbating existing allergies. "Understanding your genetic makeup can be crucial in managing food allergies and optimizing your diet for health and wellness," states Dr. El-Sohemy (El-Sohemy, 2015).

Incorporating nutrigenomic analysis for allergies into dietary planning represents a biohack that leverages genetic insights for personalized nutrition. This approach exemplifies the principle of using advanced scientific methods to tailor dietary choices to individual genetic profiles, potentially improving health outcomes and quality of life. Nutrigenomic analysis for allergies offers a cutting-edge method for customizing diet plans, aligning with the broader trend of personalized medicine and nutrition in health optimization.

Binaural Beats for Anxiety Reduction: Use auditory therapy for stress relief.

Binaural Beats for Anxiety Reduction, a technique widely embraced in the biohacking community, involves listening to audio tracks that play slightly different frequency tones in each ear, creating a perceived third tone known as a binaural beat. This auditory illusion is believed to influence brainwave patterns and can be used as a tool for stress and anxiety relief. Dr. Gerald Oster, who contributed significantly to the understanding of binaural beats, explains, "Binaural beats can induce states of relaxation, meditation, and even sleep, which is beneficial for reducing anxiety" (Oster, 1973). Oster's research indicates the potential of binaural beats in influencing the brain's electrical activity.

When listened to with headphones, binaural beats create an auditory experience that can lead the brain to a more relaxed state, corresponding to slower brainwave patterns like theta and alpha waves. This state of relaxation can help alleviate symptoms of anxiety. "The use of binaural beats for anxiety reduction is based on the brain's tendency to shift its dominant EEG frequency towards the frequency of a dominant auditory stimulus," notes Dr. Oster (Oster, 1973).

Utilizing binaural beats for anxiety reduction is a biohack that employs non-invasive, auditory stimuli to promote mental well-being. This approach aligns with the biohacking ethos of using scientifically-backed, alternative methods to enhance health and well-being. Binaural beats represent a simple yet effective tool for those seeking natural ways to manage stress and anxiety, providing a means to achieve calmness and relaxation through auditory therapy.

Hormone Optimization Therapy: Balance hormones for better health and vitality.

Hormone Optimization Therapy, an approach increasingly popular in the biohacking community, focuses on balancing hormones to improve overall health and vitality. Hormones, which are crucial regulators of many bodily processes, can become imbalanced due to factors like aging, stress, and lifestyle choices. Dr. Thierry Hertoghe, a physician specializing in hormone therapy, explains, "Optimizing hormone levels can lead to increased energy, improved mood, better muscle strength, and overall enhanced well-being" (Hertoghe, 2016). Hertoghe's insights highlight the comprehensive impact of hormone balance on health.

This therapy involves assessing individual hormonal needs and administering treatments such as bioidentical hormones to correct imbalances. Common areas of focus include thyroid hormones, testosterone, estrogen, progesterone, and cortisol. "Balancing hormones requires a personalized approach, as each individual's hormonal needs are unique," states Dr. Hertoghe (Hertoghe, 2016).

Implementing Hormone Optimization Therapy as a biohack involves careful monitoring and management of hormone levels, often under the guidance of specialized healthcare professionals. This approach is grounded in the principle of using targeted interventions to enhance bodily functions and quality of life. Hormone Optimization Therapy represents a proactive strategy for maintaining health and vitality, emphasizing the crucial role of hormones in overall physical and mental well-being.

DIY Biomechanical Analysis: Use tech for self-analysis of movement to prevent injury.

DIY Biomechanical Analysis, a method growing in popularity within the biohacking community, involves using technology to conduct self-analysis of body movements to enhance performance and prevent injury. This approach employs wearable devices, apps, and video analysis tools to gather data on how the body moves during various activities. Dr. Kelly Starrett, a physical therapist and author known for his work in human biomechanics, states, "Self-analysis of movement can identify biomechanical inefficiencies and imbalances, helping to prevent injury and improve physical performance" (Starrett, 2013). Starrett's work underscores the importance of understanding and optimizing movement patterns.

With DIY biomechanical analysis, individuals can monitor aspects such as gait, posture, and joint angles during physical activities like running, lifting, or cycling. Wearable devices can provide real-time feedback on movement quality, while video analysis software can help in visualizing and refining technique. "Using technology to analyze movement can empower individuals to make adjustments that lead to better athletic performance and reduced risk of injury," explains Dr. Starrett (Starrett, 2013).

Incorporating DIY biomechanical analysis into a fitness or health routine represents a biohack that leverages technology for self-improvement and injury prevention. This approach aligns with the biohacking ethos of using data-driven methods to enhance bodily function and performance. DIY biomechanical analysis provides a means for individuals to take an active role in understanding and improving their movement patterns, promoting better physical health and efficiency.

Nutrient IV Drips: Receive essential nutrients directly through intravenous therapy.

Nutrient IV Drips, a practice increasingly popular in the biohacking community, involve the direct infusion of essential nutrients, such as vitamins, minerals, and amino acids, into the bloodstream via intravenous therapy. This method is believed to enhance nutrient absorption by bypassing the digestive system. Dr. John Myers, who pioneered the use of intravenous vitamins and minerals, known as the Myers' Cocktail, suggests, "IV nutrient therapy can be more effective than oral supplements for correcting intracellular nutrient deficits" (Myers, 1984). His approach underlines the efficiency of IV nutrient delivery in addressing deficiencies and boosting overall health.

These nutrient IV drips can be customized to address specific health needs or goals, such as boosting energy levels, enhancing immune function, or aiding in recovery from intense physical activity. The direct infusion into the bloodstream ensures that higher concentrations of nutrients are delivered to the body's cells more efficiently than oral supplements. "Nutrient IV therapy can provide a quick and potent way to replenish essential vitamins and minerals, enhancing overall well-being," states Dr. Myers (Myers, 1984).

Incorporating Nutrient IV Drips into a wellness routine is a biohack that focuses on optimizing health at the cellular level. This approach aligns with the biohacking principle of using advanced methods to enhance bodily functions and performance. Nutrient IV therapy represents a direct and effective way to address nutrient deficiencies and promote health and vitality, offering a targeted solution for individuals seeking to boost their nutritional status.

Ecotherapy: Spend time in nature to improve mental health.

Ecotherapy, a concept widely embraced in the biohacking community, involves spending time in nature as a way to improve mental health and well-being. This practice, also known as nature therapy or green therapy, is based on the principle that direct contact with nature has significant healing properties. Dr. Ming Kuo, a researcher in environmental psychology, explains, "Exposure to natural environments can reduce stress, enhance mood, and boost cognitive functioning" (Kuo, 2015). Her research highlights the numerous psychological benefits of interacting with natural settings.

Activities under the umbrella of ecotherapy include walking in a forest, gardening, or simply spending time in a park. These activities are believed to decrease cortisol levels, the body's stress hormone, and increase feelings of relaxation and happiness. "Nature has a calming and rejuvenating effect on the mind and body, which can be especially beneficial in our fast-paced, urbanized lives," notes Dr. Kuo (Kuo, 2015).

Incorporating ecotherapy into one's routine is a biohack that utilizes the therapeutic effects of the natural environment. This approach aligns with the biohacking principle of leveraging natural, accessible resources to improve mental and physical health. Ecotherapy represents a simple yet effective way to enhance well-being, highlighting the inherent connection between humans and nature for holistic health.

Biohacking Eye Health: Implement exercises and nutrition for vision improvement.

Biohacking Eye Health, a focus within the biohacking community, involves implementing specific exercises and nutritional strategies to improve vision and overall eye health. This approach is based on the understanding that, like other parts of the body, the eyes can benefit significantly from targeted exercises and proper nutrition. Dr. William Bates, an ophthalmologist known for developing natural vision improvement techniques, states, "Regular eye exercises and proper nutrition can contribute to better vision and may help delay the onset of common eye conditions" (Bates, 1920). Bates' work underscores the potential of non-invasive methods in maintaining and enhancing eye health.

Eye health exercises can include practices such as focusing on different distances, eye tracking, and relaxation techniques to reduce eye strain and improve vision acuity. Nutritionally, incorporating foods rich in vitamins A, C, E, and minerals like zinc, along with omega-3 fatty acids, can support eye health. "Antioxidants and specific nutrients can protect against age-related degenerative eye diseases and support overall eye function," explains Dr. Bates (Bates, 1920).

Incorporating eye health exercises and nutrition into daily routines is a biohack that focuses on the proactive maintenance and improvement of vision. This approach aligns with the biohacking ethos of using natural, scientifically-backed methods to enhance bodily functions.

Biohacking eye health represents a holistic and integrative approach to vision care, emphasizing the importance of lifestyle and dietary choices in maintaining eye health and function.

Neuromodulation Devices: Use devices to alter nerve activity for pain relief and mood enhancement.

Neuromodulation Devices, increasingly popular in the biohacking community, involve using specialized devices that alter nerve activity to provide pain relief and enhance mood. These devices work by delivering electrical or magnetic stimulation to specific areas of the nervous system, thereby modulating neural activity. Dr. Norman Shealy, a neurosurgeon and a pioneer in the field of pain and stress management, notes, "Neuromodulation can effectively manage chronic pain and improve mood disorders by altering nerve impulses" (Shealy, 2008). Shealy's insights highlight the therapeutic potential of neuromodulation in treating various conditions.

Common forms of neuromodulation include Transcranial Magnetic Stimulation (TMS) for depression and spinal cord stimulation for chronic pain. These technologies offer non-pharmacological alternatives for managing pain and mood disorders. "TMS, in particular, has shown significant efficacy in treating major depressive disorders, especially in cases where traditional treatments have failed," states Dr. Shealy (Shealy, 2008).

Incorporating neuromodulation devices into a health and wellness routine represents a biohack that leverages advanced technology to enhance neurological function and well-being. This approach aligns with the biohacking principle of utilizing cutting-edge scientific methods and tools to improve quality of life. Neuromodulation devices offer a promising avenue for those seeking alternative treatments for pain management and mood enhancement, embodying a modern approach to health care and personal well-being optimization.

Mitochondrial Optimization: Focus on cellular health for energy and longevity.

Mitochondrial Optimization, a concept gaining significant attention in the biohacking community, focuses on enhancing the health and function of mitochondria – the energy-producing organelles in cells – for improved energy levels and longevity. Mitochondria play a crucial role in energy metabolism and cellular health, and their dysfunction is linked to aging and various chronic diseases. Dr. Douglas Wallace, a geneticist specializing in mitochondrial biology, explains, "Optimizing mitochondrial function can have profound effects on energy levels and lifespan, as mitochondria are critical for energy production and metabolic processes" (Wallace, 2010). His research underscores the importance of mitochondrial health for overall well-being.

Strategies for mitochondrial optimization include a nutrient-rich diet, regular exercise, intermittent fasting, and reducing exposure to toxins. Nutrients such as CoQ10, magnesium, and omega-3 fatty acids are particularly important for mitochondrial function. "A lifestyle that supports mitochondrial health can lead to improved energy utilization and potentially slow down the aging process," states Dr. Wallace (Wallace, 2010).

Adopting a mitochondrial optimization strategy is a biohack that focuses on the cellular level to enhance overall health and vitality. This approach is aligned with the biohacking ethos of using science-based methods to improve bodily functions. Mitochondrial optimization represents a comprehensive approach to health maintenance, emphasizing the foundational role of cellular energy in physical and mental performance.

Posture Correction Devices: Utilize wearable tech to improve posture.

Posture Correction Devices, increasingly popular in the biohacking community, involve the use of wearable technology to improve posture and alleviate related discomforts. These devices are designed to detect and correct poor posture by providing real-time feedback, often through vibrations or auditory signals, prompting the user to adjust their posture. Dr. Steven Weiniger, a posture expert and author, explains, "Maintaining good posture is essential for musculoskeletal health, and posture correction devices can be effective tools in building awareness and correcting postural habits" (Weiniger, 2016). Weiniger's insights highlight the importance of posture in overall health and well-being.

These devices typically work by being attached to the body or clothing, monitoring spinal alignment and body position throughout the day. When poor posture is detected, the device alerts the user, encouraging immediate correction. This constant feedback loop helps in training the muscles to maintain proper alignment. "Posture correction devices can aid in reducing back pain, improving breathing, and enhancing physical appearance," states Dr. Weiniger (Weiniger, 2016).

Incorporating posture correction devices into daily life is a biohack that leverages technology to improve physical health. This approach aligns with the biohacking principle of using data-driven tools to enhance bodily functions. Posture correction devices represent a practical and effective method to address the widespread issue of poor posture, especially prevalent in today's sedentary lifestyle, offering a pathway to better health and comfort.

Hyperbaric Oxygen Therapy: Use increased atmospheric pressure to enhance oxygen absorption.

Hyperbaric Oxygen Therapy (HBOT), a technique embraced by the biohacking community, involves breathing pure oxygen in a pressurized room or chamber. This therapy is based on the principle that under increased atmospheric pressure, the body can absorb more oxygen than under normal conditions. Dr. Paul Harch, a leading expert in hyperbaric medicine, explains, "Hyperbaric oxygen therapy saturates the body's tissues with high levels of oxygen, which can accelerate healing processes, reduce inflammation, and improve brain function" (Harch, 2017). Harch's insights underscore the wide-ranging therapeutic potential of HBOT.

In an HBOT chamber, the air pressure is increased to up to three times higher than normal air pressure. Under these conditions, the lungs can gather more oxygen than would be possible breathing pure oxygen at normal air pressure. This extra oxygen can help fight bacteria and stimulate the release of growth factors and stem cells, which promote healing. "HBOT has been successfully used to treat conditions like decompression sickness, serious infections, and wounds that won't heal as a result of diabetes or radiation injury," notes Dr. Harch (Harch, 2017).

Adopting HBOT as a biohack involves utilizing this therapy to enhance overall health and well-being, particularly in the areas of recovery and healing. This approach aligns with the biohacking ethos of exploring advanced medical therapies to optimize body functions. HBOT represents a unique and effective treatment method, offering benefits for a range of health conditions and enhancing the body's natural healing processes.

Magnet Therapy: Investigate the potential benefits of magnetic fields on body processes.

Magnet Therapy, a practice that has garnered interest within the biohacking community, involves the use of magnetic fields to potentially influence various body processes for therapeutic benefits. This approach is based on the belief that magnetic fields can affect bodily functions, leading to improved health and wellness. Dr. William Pawluk, a former Johns Hopkins University physician and an expert in medical magnet therapy, explains, "Magnetic fields can have a profound effect on the body, potentially improving circulation, reducing inflammation, and promoting tissue healing" (Pawluk, 2010). Pawluk's insights highlight the potential therapeutic applications of magnetic fields.

Magnet therapy typically involves the application of static or pulsed magnetic fields through various devices, including magnetic bracelets, insoles, and mattresses. The theory behind this therapy is that these fields can penetrate the body and influence cellular function, leading to improved health outcomes. "While the exact mechanisms are still being studied, evidence suggests that magnetic therapy can have a beneficial effect on the body, particularly in pain management and wound healing," states Dr. Pawluk (Pawluk, 2010).

Incorporating magnet therapy into a wellness routine is a biohack that explores the influence of magnetic fields on physical health. This approach aligns with the biohacking principle of using non-invasive, alternative therapies to enhance well-being. Magnet therapy represents an area of interest for those seeking to explore the potential health benefits of magnetic fields, offering a novel approach to pain relief and overall health enhancement.

Laser Therapy for Tissue Repair: Use low-level lasers for healing and pain relief.

Laser Therapy for Tissue Repair, increasingly adopted in the biohacking community, involves the use of low-level lasers (or cold lasers) to stimulate healing and provide pain relief. This non-invasive therapy uses specific wavelengths of light to interact with tissue, accelerating the healing process by increasing blood flow and stimulating cellular repair. Dr. James Carroll, a foremost expert in photobiomodulation (low-level laser therapy), explains, "Low-level laser therapy can promote tissue repair and reduce inflammation and pain in a range of conditions, from musculoskeletal injuries to chronic disorders" (Carroll, 2012). Carroll's insights underscore the therapeutic potential of laser therapy in tissue healing and pain management.

The therapy works by emitting photons, which are absorbed by the mitochondria in cells, leading to increased production of adenosine triphosphate (ATP), and, subsequently, enhanced cellular metabolism. This process can reduce inflammation, alleviate pain, and accelerate tissue repair. "Laser therapy has been shown to be effective in accelerating the healing process in injuries, reducing pain in chronic conditions, and improving functionality and quality of life," states Dr. Carroll (Carroll, 2012).

Incorporating laser therapy for tissue repair into a health and wellness routine is a biohack that leverages advanced light technology to enhance the body's natural healing processes. This approach aligns with the biohacking ethos of using science-backed, non-invasive methods for health optimization. Laser therapy represents a promising tool for those seeking effective, drug-free alternatives for pain relief and tissue healing, offering a modern approach to managing health and well-being.

Biometric Mood Tracking: Monitor physiological indicators to understand and manage emotions.

Biometric Mood Tracking, a practice gaining traction in the biohacking community, involves monitoring physiological indicators such as heart rate variability (HRV), skin conductance, and brainwave patterns to understand and manage emotions. This method leverages wearable technology and sensors to provide real-time data about the body's physical responses, which can be correlated with emotional states. Dr. Rosalind Picard, a researcher in affective computing at MIT, explains, "By tracking physiological changes, we can gain insights into our emotional reactions and learn to better manage our emotional health" (Picard, 2015). Picard's research emphasizes the connection between physiological signals and emotional states.

Biometric mood tracking devices can help identify patterns of stress, relaxation, and emotional arousal. This information can be incredibly valuable for individuals seeking to understand their emotional triggers and improve emotional regulation. For example, a sudden increase in HRV might indicate stress or anxiety, prompting the user to employ stress-relief techniques. "Understanding your body's responses to different emotions can lead to more effective strategies for emotional management and well-being," notes Dr. Picard (Picard, 2015).

Incorporating biometric mood tracking into daily life is a biohack that utilizes the latest in wearable technology to enhance emotional intelligence and mental health. This approach aligns with the biohacking principle of using data-driven tools to gain deeper insights into one's health and well-being. Biometric mood tracking offers a sophisticated and proactive way to manage emotional health, representing a convergence of technology, psychology, and self-care.

Kinesiology Tape for Muscle Support: Apply therapeutic tape for injury prevention and support.

Kinesiology Tape for Muscle Support, a method widely used in the biohacking and athletic communities, involves the application of a special elastic therapeutic tape on the skin to provide support for muscles and joints, aiding in injury prevention and recovery. The tape is designed to mimic the skin's elasticity, allowing for a full range of motion while still providing support and stability. Dr. Kenzo Kase, a chiropractor and the creator of the original Kinesio Tape, explains, "Kinesiology tape can help reduce pain and inflammation, support muscles, and enhance performance without restricting movement" (Kase, 1979). Kase's insights highlight the tape's versatility and effectiveness in supporting muscular function.

Kinesiology tape works by gently lifting the skin, creating a small space between the muscle and dermis layers. This space is believed to improve blood and lymph circulation, reduce swelling and inflammation, and facilitate faster healing. "The tape can also provide sensory feedback to the body, which helps in maintaining proper posture and alignment," adds Dr. Kase (Kase, 1979).

Incorporating kinesiology tape into a fitness or rehabilitation routine is a biohack that leverages the physical and neurological benefits of this unique taping method. This approach is aligned with the biohacking ethos of using innovative, non-invasive methods to enhance physical health and performance. Kinesiology tape represents a practical tool for athletes, fitness enthusiasts, and anyone seeking additional muscle and joint support, offering a simple yet effective solution for improved movement and injury prevention.

Lymphatic Drainage Techniques: Use massage and exercises to enhance lymphatic system function.

Lymphatic Drainage Techniques, increasingly adopted by the biohacking community, involve specific massage methods and exercises designed to enhance the function of the lymphatic system, a critical part of the body's immune and waste-removal systems. This approach helps in the movement of lymph, a fluid that carries waste products away from tissues, back towards the heart. Dr.

Bruno Chikly, a physician known for his work in lymphatic therapy, states, "Lymphatic drainage techniques can significantly improve the efficiency of the lymphatic system, helping to detoxify the body, reduce swelling, and boost immune function" (Chikly, 2001). Chikly's research underscores the health benefits of maintaining an efficient lymphatic system.

Lymphatic drainage techniques typically involve gentle, rhythmic massage that follows the direction of lymph flow. This method is believed to stimulate the movement of lymph through its vessels, aiding in the removal of waste products and excess fluid from body tissues. Additionally, specific exercises and stretching can also support lymph flow. "These techniques not only help in reducing lymphedema but also play a role in detoxification and enhancing overall well-being," explains Dr. Chikly (Chikly, 2001).

Implementing lymphatic drainage techniques as a biohack is an approach that focuses on supporting the body's natural detoxification processes. This method aligns with the biohacking ethos of using non-invasive, natural techniques to enhance bodily functions. Lymphatic drainage represents a powerful tool for health maintenance and recovery, offering benefits like improved immune function and reduced inflammation, making it an integral part of a holistic health and wellness routine.

Voice Analysis for Health Monitoring: Analyze voice patterns for signs of health issues.

Voice Analysis for Health Monitoring, a practice gaining momentum in the biohacking and medical communities, involves analyzing voice patterns to detect potential health issues. This approach is based on the idea that changes in voice characteristics can be indicative of various health conditions, ranging from mood disorders to neurological diseases. Dr. Rita Singh, a researcher in voice forensics, explains, "Voice analysis can provide insights into a person's health, as changes in voice qualities can reflect underlying medical conditions" (Singh, 2018). Singh's work highlights the potential of voice analysis as a non-invasive diagnostic tool.

Advancements in AI and machine learning have enabled the development of algorithms that can analyze subtle qualities in a person's voice, such as tone, pitch, and cadence. These analyses can potentially reveal signs of stress, depression, Parkinson's disease, and even heart conditions. "The voice is not just a medium of communication; it can also be a telltale sign of your health and well-being," notes Dr. Singh (Singh, 2018).

Incorporating voice analysis into health monitoring represents a biohack that leverages cutting-edge technology to enhance personal health awareness. This approach is aligned with the biohacking principle of using data-driven methods for early detection and management of health conditions. Voice analysis for health monitoring offers a unique, non-invasive way to potentially identify and address health issues, demonstrating the growing intersection of technology and healthcare in personal health management.

Personal Air Quality Monitors: Track exposure to pollutants for respiratory health.

Personal Air Quality Monitors, increasingly used in the biohacking community, are devices designed to track exposure to various pollutants in the environment to protect and improve respiratory health. These monitors measure factors like particulate matter, volatile organic compounds (VOCs), carbon dioxide, and other harmful pollutants in the air. Dr. Maria Neira, a public health expert at the World Health Organization, emphasizes the importance of monitoring air quality, stating, "Being aware of the air quality in your immediate environment can help you reduce your exposure to harmful pollutants and lower the risk of respiratory diseases" (Neira, 2017). Neira's insights underscore the significance of air quality on overall health.

Personal air quality monitors can be portable or stationary and often link to smartphone apps, providing real-time data on air quality. This information can be crucial for individuals with respiratory conditions like asthma or allergies, as well as those living in urban areas with high pollution levels. "Understanding the air quality in your surroundings can inform decisions about outdoor activities, ventilation, and the use of air purifiers," explains Dr. Neira (Neira, 2017).

Incorporating personal air quality monitors into daily life is a biohack that aligns with the proactive management of health in relation to environmental factors. This approach exemplifies the biohacking ethos of using technology to gather data for health optimization. Personal air quality monitors represent a practical tool for those seeking to minimize their exposure to air pollutants, highlighting the importance of environmental factors in maintaining good health and well-being.

Conclusion

As we conclude our exploration of the diverse and innovative world of biohacking, it's clear that this field represents a confluence of science, technology, and a profound commitment to personal well-being. Throughout this book, we've delved into various biohacking strategies, from the simple and natural to the technologically advanced, each offering unique ways to enhance health, longevity, and overall quality of life.

Biohacking, at its core, is about empowerment and personalization. It encourages us to take control of our own health by understanding our unique biological makeup and leveraging cutting-edge scientific research. The techniques we've explored, ranging from nutritional tweaks and exercise regimens to advanced therapies like gene editing and neurofeedback, showcase the vast potential of biohacking. They underline a crucial truth: that the pursuit of health and well-being is as diverse and individualized as we are.

Moreover, this book underscores the importance of a holistic approach to health. Biohacking isn't just about optimizing physical health; it also encompasses mental and emotional well-being. The integration of various methods – be it mindfulness practices, stress management techniques, or mood-enhancing strategies – highlights the interconnectedness of different aspects of health.

As biohacking continues to evolve, driven by technological advancements and deeper scientific understanding, its potential grows. However, it's important to approach biohacking with mindfulness, balancing enthusiasm with caution, and always prioritizing safety and ethical considerations.

Biohacking empowers us to be architects of our own health, encouraging a proactive, informed, and holistic approach to living our best lives. It is a testament to human ingenuity and the unyielding pursuit of personal excellence and well-being. As you apply the insights from this book, remember that the journey of biohacking is deeply personal and constantly evolving – a pursuit of balance, health, and vitality that is as unique as each of us.